Contents

Preface

Prostate cancer is rare in men before the age of 40. However, by the time they reach 80, some 80% of men may have prostate cancer, although in many cases it does not cause any symptoms and remains clinically undetected, death eventually being due to other, unrelated, causes. Most prostate cancers are quite slow growing, although in some men - for reasons that remain unclear - they can progress more rapidly.

The causes of prostate cancer are not yet understood, but it is known to have an ethnic association. Until recently, the highest rate of the disease was thought to occur amongst black American men in the USA, but a study has now shown the incidence in Jamaica to be even higher. In contrast, prostate cancer is relatively rare amongst American Indians, Hispanics and Orientals, such as the Chinese and Japanese. There is also evidence that it has a genetic basis - men with a first-degree relative with prostate cancer having a greater risk than normal of developing the disease.

This book provides up-to-date, clear explanations of what is currently known about prostate cancer. It describes the treatments that are available, as well as the different types of complementary therapies, and discusses possible risk factors and the potential role of diet in the development of the disease.

Jane Smith
Raj Persad
Kieran Jefferson
Biral Patel

Chapter 1

Introduction

There are various problems that can affect the prostate gland, but before discussing these, it is useful to have some understanding of the structure and function of the male reproductive organs.

The male reproductive organs

The urethra is the tube in both men and women that drains urine from the bladder. In men it also carries the semen that is ejaculated following sexual arousal. The male urethra is about 20 cm (8 inches) long and extends from the neck of the bladder to the tip of the penis.

In a male fetus, two testes (or testicles) develop near the kidneys, but by birth they have normally descended through a canal in the abdominal wall and into the scrotum. Each of the testes is an oval, glandular organ, about 4 cm (1.5 inches) long by 2.5 cm (1 inch) wide, which contains the seminiferous tubules that produce sperm. The sperm pass down a system of ducts and tubes into the two seminal vesicles, which lie at the base of the bladder next to the prostate gland. When ejaculation occurs, large numbers of sperm, together with secretions from the prostate, are pumped from the seminal vesicles into the urethra as semen, and the muscle in the neck of the bladder contracts to prevent the semen passing back into it.

The prostate gland

The prostate gland is normally about the size and shape of a walnut. It is partly enclosed in a capsule of muscle and connective tissue and its surface is covered with blood vessels and nerves. A furrow running down its centre divides it into a left and right lobe. Because the urethra runs

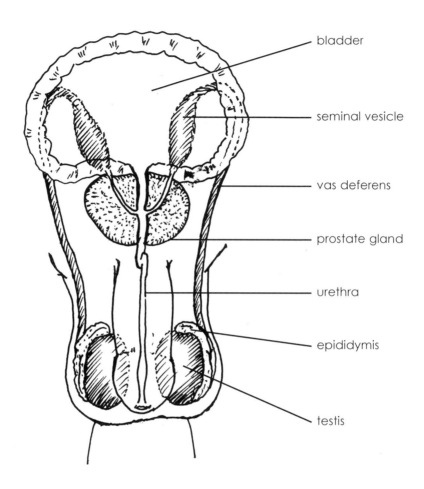

The male genital system.

bladder

seminal vesicle

vas deferens

prostate gland

urethra

epididymis

testis

through the prostate gland, problems that affect the prostate often make it difficult to pass urine.

The precise function of the prostate is not fully understood, but it is believed to secrete a fluid that contributes to the fertility of sperm.

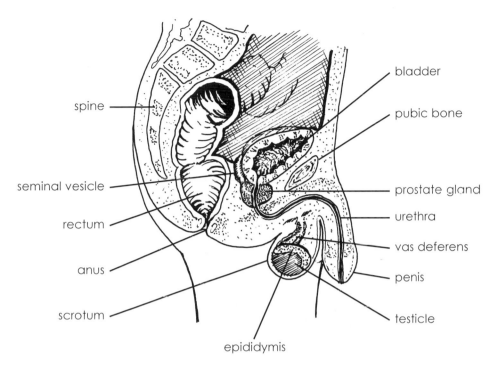

spine

seminal vesicle

rectum

anus

scrotum

epididymis

bladder

pubic bone

prostate gland

urethra

vas deferens

penis

testicle

The male reproductive system.

Both the growth and function of the prostate gland are regulated by a complex interaction of numerous steroid and other hormones, but mainly by the male sex hormone testosterone, which is produced by the testes. With age, the hormonal regulation tends to break down and the prostate gland enlarges. This enlargement may cause symptoms, the severity of which is not directly related to the size of the prostate.

There are three main types of prostate problem:

❖   benign enlargement of the prostate gland (benign prostatic hyperplasia), which is a normal, age-related change that can cause minor or more troublesome urinary symptoms;

❖   inflammation of the prostate gland (called prostatitis);

❖   prostate cancer.

Benign prostatic hyperplasia and prostatitis are not cancers and are therefore dealt with only briefly (see Chapter 2).

Prostate cancer

What is a cancer?

The human body is made up of an incomprehensibly large number of cells, which are only visible under a microscope. These cells are organized into tissues, which themselves form organs, each of which has a specific function. For the organs to function effectively and for a person to remain healthy, the proportions and functions of each type of cell within the tissues must be controlled. Cell number is controlled by regulation of the division and survival of individual cells. Uncontrolled division of a single cell can produce a swelling known as a tumour. Tumours can be benign (non-cancerous) or malignant (a cancer).

Myth
Once you've got prostate cancer, there's no real cure.

Truth
Prostate cancer can be cured if it's caught early enough. There are also good treatments that can delay the progression of most incurable prostate cancers. However, some prostate cancers do not need aggressive treatment because they are not likely to cause any harm to men who have them.

Although benign tumours can cause pain and interfere with the normal function of nearby organs as they grow, they are rarely life threatening, usually respond to treatment and do not spread to other parts of the body. Malignant tumours, on the other hand, destroy nearby cells as they grow, and their own cells can break off and be carried in the blood or lymphatic vessels to other parts of the body. This process of spread is known as metastasis and the secondary tumours that result from it are called metastases. A biopsy can be done to remove a small sample of the cells of a tumour, which is then examined under a microscope to see if the cells are benign or malignant.

The lymphatic vessels contain lymph, a clear fluid that drains excess cells, protein and fluid away from the tissues. As the lymph passes through glands (called lymph nodes) at various sites around the body, some of the substances in it, including any cancer cells, are filtered out, which is why cancers often spread first to the lymph nodes closest to them.

Symptoms

A small prostate cancer may not cause any symptoms and may even remain undetected during rectal examination (see page 32). In fact, prostate cancers often only come to light because testing reveals a raised level of prostate-specific antigen (PSA, see page 33). As a prostate tumour grows, it can cause difficulty urinating, although it should be stressed that this is more commonly a symptom of other, non-cancerous, conditions such as benign prostatic hyperplasia (see page 8).

Prostate cancer tends to spread to the lymph nodes and bones, especially those of the hip and lower back, and bone pain is therefore sometimes an indication that the disease has spread. Tests can be done to detect the stage of development of a prostate cancer, and treatment is more likely to be successful if it is carried out at an early stage before spread has occurred.

Incidence

In the UK, approximately 20,000 men are newly diagnosed as having prostate cancer each year. Adenocarcinoma of the prostate (cancer of the glandular epithelium) is the most common male cancer in the UK. Most of those affected are elderly, but an increasing number of prostate cancers are being diagnosed in young and middle-aged men in their forties and fifties.

> **Myth**
> Only old men get prostate cancer.
>
> **Truth**
> Although prostate cancer is much more common in older men, it is a significant cause of illness in men after the age of 50.

Although many prostate cancers are relatively harmless and there has been confusion about the treatment of older men with the disease, it is now clear that about 20% of men with prostate cancer die from the disease (which compares closely with the figure of 25% of women with breast cancer).

The incidence of prostate cancer has risen steadily throughout the world during the past 25 years. In some countries at least, this may be linked to the increased use of tests - such as that for PSA (see page 33) - detecting cases that would previously have gone unnoticed, although this cannot be the whole explanation and other possible reasons include increased public awareness about the disease and a growing elderly population.

The incidence of prostate cancer varies considerably in men of different races and in different countries. It is believed to be common in men of Northern European races and rare in Asian men. Certain high-risk groups have been identified, including men from the Caribbean. However, interestingly, the incidence of latent disease (i.e. disease that only shows up on post-mortem examination and has not been the cause of death) does not vary between populations. Autopsy data from various countries indicate that 15-30% of men above the age of 50 have latent prostate cancer, but it is not yet clear whether this represents an early stage of the disease or is different from the prostate cancer that is detected clinically. It is possible that, in parts of Europe and the USA at least, the reduction seen in the number of deaths from prostate cancer may be due to improvements in the treatment of more advanced disease rather than to an increase in the detection of early cancers. Whatever the situation, it is certainly true that far fewer men die from prostate cancer than have the disease.

The risk of getting prostate cancer increases in men who emigrate from a country where the incidence is low to one where it is high. For example, Japanese migrants to the USA have a much higher risk of disease compared to native Japanese men. The role of race in the incidence of prostate cancer is discussed in more detail in Chapter 3.

Chapter 2

Benign diseases of the prostate

Many men develop prostate problems as they get older, most of which are due to benign conditions rather than cancer. This chapter deals briefly with the non-cancerous diseases that can affect the prostate gland.

Benign prostatic hyperplasia

This condition results in an age-related enlargement of the prostate gland and is most common in men over 50, although growth of (and microscopic changes in) the prostate may begin around the age of 30, and there is a phase of accelerated growth around 40. About 50% of men have benign prostatic hyperplasia by the time they are 60.

Symptoms

As the prostate gland grows, it can constrict and block the urethra, causing a variety of urinary symptoms. However, the degree of obstruction is not necessarily directly related to the size of the prostate, but may be partly dependent on the tone (elasticity) of the prostatic muscles and muscles in the neck of the bladder.

The syndrome caused by benign prostatic hyperplasia is often called prostatism. It involves symptoms of urinary obstruction, such as a decreased or hesitant flow of urine and a feeling of incomplete emptying of the bladder. Symptoms of irritation may also occur if the bladder muscles have to work harder to overcome the obstruction. These irritative symptoms include a sudden urge to urinate and a need to urinate frequently during the night. Similar symptoms may also be associated with various other conditions. In a small number of cases, complications such as acute or chronic urine retention can develop if the symptoms remain untreated (see page 12).

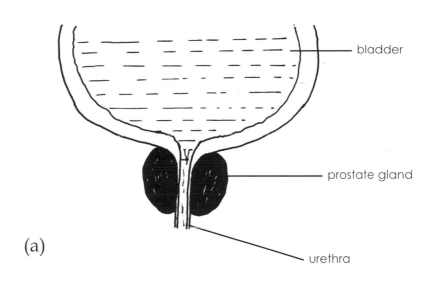

(a)

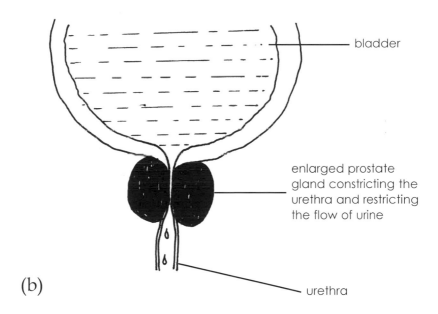

(b)

(a) A normal prostate gland *allows urine to flow freely from the bladder.*
(b) When the prostate gland is enlarged, *it constricts the urethra and blocks the flow of urine.*

Although benign prostatic hyperplasia is a progressive condition, its symptoms sometimes improve temporarily. However, if left untreated, it can result in:

❖ thickening of the muscles of the bladder wall (hypertrophy);

❖ the retention of some urine in the bladder after urination (urinary stasis), possibly leading to the build up of bacteria and to urinary tract infection, which may be recurrent and may result in cystitis and bladder stones;

❖ stretching of the tubes that drain the kidneys due to the accumulation of urine, which is sometimes a result of urinary retention and can cause 'back pressure' on the kidneys (hydronephrosis);

❖ over-activity of the muscular layers of the bladder wall (detrusor instability), leading to irritative symptoms (see above);

❖ inability of the bladder muscle to contract properly (detrusor decompensation), causing it to lose its elasticity and become weak and floppy (atonic).

Causes

The causes of benign prostatic hyperplasia are not fully understood, but it is known that its development is associated with ageing and with the testicular hormones.

Prostatitis

Prostatitis can occur in different forms, all of which tend to affect relatively young men, commonly between the ages of 20 and 50. Although prostatitis does not involve enlargement of the prostate gland, the symptoms may be similar and a transrectal ultrasound scan and biopsy (see page 34) are sometimes useful to help diagnose the condition. Classification systems vary, but a simplified system is given below.

National Institutes of Health classification of prostatitis

Category	Name	Description
I	Acute bacterial prostatitis	Acute infection of the prostate gland
II	Chronic bacterial prostatitis	Recurrent urinary tract infection; chronic infection of the prostate
III	Chronic abacterial prostatitis/ chronic pelvic pain syndrome	Discomfort or pain in the pelvic region; variable voiding and sexual symptoms; no demonstrable infection
IIIA	Inflammatory chronic pelvic pain syndrome	Excessive number of white cells in semen
IIIB	Non-inflammatory pelvic pain syndrome	Insignificant number of white cells in semen
IV	Asymptomatic inflammatory prostatitis	Evidence of inflammation in biopsy/semen; no symptoms

Bacterial prostatitis

Bacterial prostatitis can be acute, with symptoms similar to those of urinary infection: pain when passing urine, bladder pain, fever and frequent urination. There is also a chronic form of the infection, the symptoms of which are sometimes brought on by bowel motions, tend to recur and may include back pain, discomfort around the lower abdomen and genitals, and pain when passing urine. A sample of the bacteria in the urine can be grown in a laboratory so that they can be identified and the appropriate antibiotic selected for treatment.

Abacterial prostatitis

Abacterial prostatitis has symptoms similar to the bacterial form but which tend to come and go and can be fairly vague. They include discomfort around the genitals, between the scrotum and anus (the area known as the perineum), in the lower abdomen and low back. However, no bacteria can be found in the urine or prostatic fluid. Treatment with a long course of antibiotics is sometimes successful. Although it is a chronic condition, which can be difficult to clear up completely, treatment of the symptoms is often all that can be done.

Prostatodynia

Prostatodynia means prostate pain. Its cause is difficult to identify and often the only course of action available is to treat its symptoms.

Other causes of urinary problems

Some of the conditions described below can be associated with prostate disease, although all of them can have other causes.

Urine retention

As well as sometimes being caused by prostate problems, urine retention can also be due, for example, to a prolapsed vertebral disc, any type of operation or constipation.

Acute urine retention may develop suddenly and be accompanied by pain. It can occur in the early stages of a prostate condition because of constipation or voluntarily retaining urine, for example when you need to urinate but are unable to get to a toilet. The initial treatment is to insert a catheter (see page 31) through the penis or through a small cut made in the skin above the pubic bone (suprapubically). If urine retention is due to something other than enlargement of the prostate, the catheter can be removed as soon as urine can be passed spontaneously. When it is due to benign prostate enlargement, an operation may be necessary to reduce the size of the prostate gland and enable bladder control to be regained, if treatment with drugs is unsuccessful or the symptoms are severe.

Chronic urine retention occurs when the bladder is unable to empty completely over a period of time. It does not cause pain, but there may be symptoms such as incontinence and dribbling of urine after urination. The abdomen may swell as the bladder enlarges, and trouser waistbands may become noticeably tighter. If this situation continues for some time, the build-up of pressure may eventually affect the kidneys. Although in its early stages kidney failure usually has no symptoms, it eventually leads to a general feeling of being unwell and may cause weight loss.

The treatment of chronic urine retention sometimes involves a period of catheterization (see page 30) to try to improve kidney function, and surgery may be necessary before the catheter can be removed.

Atonic bladder

The symptoms of an atonic bladder are often similar to those of chronic urine retention: a full bladder, difficulty passing urine and possibly incontinence. The condition occurs when the bladder fills up and the muscle of its wall loses its ability to contract and squeeze out the urine efficiently, which eventually causes the bladder to become a floppy sac.

Surgery to reduce the size of an enlarged prostate gland may not resolve the problems of an atonic bladder and, for older men with mild symptoms, treatment is often unnecessary. However, if infection develops because there is a stagnant pool of urine left in the bladder, catheterization may be required, sometimes permanently (see page 30). Most people can, if necessary, be taught the technique of intermittent self-catheterization.

Intermittent self-catheterization

To be able to perform this technique, you need to be motivated and to have a reasonable amount of manual dexterity. You will be shown how to insert a catheter to empty your bladder before it becomes full of urine. The catheters used are small and disposable and are coated with a substance that allows them to slide easily into the urethra. They are not uncomfortable or difficult to insert and have a very low rate of associated infection.

Irritable bladder

If the bladder muscle is over-active, it may cause urinary symptoms such as the frequent need to pass small amounts of urine and increased urgency, which sometimes results in the leakage of urine before a toilet can be reached. Similar symptoms can also be due to irritation of the bladder by stones or tumours. An irritable bladder that has no underlying cause can be treated with a type of drug called an anticholinergic, which is given as tablets and acts on the nerves to the bladder. However, over-activity of the bladder muscles can also be due to obstruction by an enlarged prostate gland.

Urethral stricture

Although narrowing of the urethra may have no obvious cause, in the past it was often the result of physical damage, for example following an accident, or of infection such as gonorrhoea. However, it is now more likely to occur after surgery, including transurethral resection of the prostate, or catheterization (see page 30). Its symptoms include a reduced flow of urine and less powerful, more frequent urination.

Nocturnal polyuria

Normally, the action of antidiuretic hormone (which is produced by the brain) reduces the function of the kidneys at night so that they produce less urine. However, as the 'body clock' alters with age, people often need to pass large amounts of urine during the night, possibly as much as they do during daytime. This condition is known as nocturnal polyuria.

It may be helpful to drink less in the evenings, but there are drugs that might be more effective. A diuretic tablet such as frusemide can be taken in the early evening so that a lot of urine is passed before bedtime, thus reducing the amount produced during the night. Alternatively, desmopressin (an artificial analogue of antidiuretic hormone that is given as a nasal spray or tablets) can be taken just before bedtime to turn the kidneys off for the night. However, as desmopressin can cause fluid retention in people with other medical problems, its use is not always appropriate.

Chapter 3

Risk factors for prostate cancer

Until fairly recently, the only risk factors that were known to be associated with prostate cancer were age, race and family history - as well, of course, as male sex. However, other factors have now been implicated, although their association with the actual risk of developing prostate cancer remains inconclusive.

Race

Prostate cancer appears to have a genetic component and is more common in Negroes and very uncommon in people of oriental origin. However, for oriental men who move from their own country to the USA (particularly Japanese men, who have a very low risk of prostate cancer), the incidence increases, although it still remains lower than that of both American Caucasians and African-Americans. This suggests that there may be another factor involved, which could be diet - Americans eat a diet high in fats, whereas Japan has one of the lowest rates of fat consumption in the world.

The world's highest rate of prostate cancer appears to be amongst men from the Caribbean, followed by the African-American population in the USA. In the USA, African-Americans have been reported to have a 66% higher incidence of prostate cancer than Caucasians and are twice as likely to die from it. Conversely, the incidence amongst Negroes in Africa is one of the lowest in the world - although the low recorded incidence could be due to incomplete medical recording and the poor availability of health care in Africa in general.

Heredity

The risk of developing prostate cancer is greater (possibly by as much as three times) for men who have a first-degree relative (e.g. a father or brother) with the disease than it is for men without this family history. The more affected relatives a man has (particularly if they developed prostate cancer at an early age), the more likely he is to develop the disease. It is also believed that a family history of breast cancer increases the chances of a man developing prostate cancer.

Various genes have been identified (including one called the *HPC* gene) that are thought to be associated with a *susceptibility* to prostate cancer. However, the presence of these genes does not indicate a definite risk of developing the disease, and other factors are also likely to be involved. There is, as yet, no genetic test available.

Age

The concept that prostate cancer is a disease of old age is now known to be somewhat inaccurate. It is not uncommon for men to develop cancer of the prostate in their 50s or even their 40s, although it is estimated that 80% of cases are diagnosed in men over the age of 65 years. White men in the USA aged between 75 and 79 are about 130 times more likely to develop prostate cancer than those aged between 45 and 49 - an age-related increase in incidence that is greater than for any other type of cancer. However, prostate cancer is common in men aged 50-70 in all developed countries and it may be that the damage to DNA that occurs with age causes genetic alterations that may play some role in this.

Hormones

The sex hormones

The sex hormones (known as androgens), and particularly testosterone and its active form dihydrotestosterone, seem to trigger or promote prostate cancer. In many cases, the cancer regresses when androgen stimulation is removed and this is now an accepted treatment for certain forms of prostate cancer. The disease is very rare amongst men who have been castrated at an early age or who have errors of androgen metabolism.

The following hormonal factors have been suggested to play a part in increasing the risk of prostate cancer:

❖ a high testosterone to dihydrotestosterone ratio in the plasma,

❖ high levels of testosterone in the circulation,

❖ low oestrogen levels,

❖ low levels of sex-hormone binding globulin (SHBG), a hormone that binds to testosterone in the circulation and reduces its availability.

Insulin-like growth factors

Insulin-like growth factors (IGFs) play a role in cell proliferation and metabolism. Raised levels of serum IGFs are the strongest known risk factors for the subsequent development of prostate cancer in men and of breast cancer in women.

Diet

A number of studies have suggested that a diet high in vitamins D and E, vitamin A from plant sources, lycopene from tomatoes, and omega-3 fatty acids from fish oils has a protective effect (see Chapter 4), whereas eating a lot of animal fat appears to increase the risk of developing prostate cancer.

Fat, meat and dairy products

Positive links have been consistently reported between prostate cancer and fat, meat and dairy products in the diet. The particular types of fat that seem to be implicated include animal fat and both saturated and mono-unsaturated fat. It is possible - but unproven - that the fat in animal products may increase the level of the sex hormones in the body, by some means not yet identified. Studies do seem to indicate that reducing the amount of fat in the diet can slow the progression of prostate cancer in men who already have the disease.

Body size and weight

There is no proof of a direct association between obesity and the risk of prostate cancer. It is possible, however, that overweight or obese people may eat a high-fat diet and that the increased risk observed is due to this, rather than to the obesity itself.

Men who are obese have a higher level of the hormone oestrogen and a lower level of testosterone than normal, both of which might be expected to decrease the risk of prostate cancer (see above). However, studies have given conflicting results: one showed that men with a lean body mass may have an increased risk of developing the disease, whereas in another, obesity in pre-adolescence seemed to be associated with a lower risk of developing the disease in adulthood. It is possible that there is a link between androgen levels during puberty and the later development of prostate cancer.

Some studies have also indicated a link between height and prostate cancer, whereas others have failed to do so. Again, if there is such a connection, it could be associated with hormone levels during puberty and adolescence.

Smoking

There is an association between smoking and the risk of dying from prostate cancer, rather than with the incidence of the disease itself. Some studies have shown that prostate cancers are diagnosed at a later stage in smokers, although it may simply be that smokers are more likely than non-smokers to put off seeking medical attention. However, it is possible that there is an unidentified mechanism by which tobacco increases the virulence of the disease.

Occupational hazards

No single occupation has been closely linked to prostate cancer, although there is thought to be a possible weak association with exposure to cadmium (see below) and possibly also with working in a nuclear power station.

Cadmium

Zinc is essential for the replication and repair of DNA and RNA, and its concentration in the prostate gland is high. Exposure to cadmium in the welding and electroplating industries, for example, antagonizes the effect of zinc and may therefore increase the risk of prostate cancer, although the results of studies have been inconclusive.

Herbicides

Although some studies have reported a link between the use of herbicides by farmers and prostate cancer risk, if any such association does exist, it is believed to be weak.

Radiation

A slight increase in risk has been reported among the survivors of atomic bombs who have been exposed to high doses of radiation, although there is little evidence to suggest that occupational radiation exposure has any effect on prostate cancer risk.

Vasectomy

Whether or not there is an association between vasectomy and prostate cancer remains controversial. Although one study found a 50% raised risk of developing prostate cancer amongst men who had undergone a vasectomy - a risk that increased with time since the operation - the evidence for such an association has been inconsistent.

It is possible that vasectomized men have higher levels of circulating testosterone and lower levels of SHBG (see above). Vasectomy also decreases prostate secretion, which may increase the exposure of the cells of the gland to carcinogenic substances in the prostate fluid.

Chapter 4
Prevention and complementary therapies

Physical activity

Physical activity (such as walking to work) may have a slight protective effect against the risk of developing prostate cancer, although studies have proved inconclusive. It is possible that any such effect is the result of exercise altering the metabolism of the sex hormones - for example, some highly trained male athletes have been reported to have lower than normal levels of testosterone. However, there does not seem to be any equivalent connection with moderate activity levels.

Dietary factors

It seems that the risk of prostate cancer can be reduced (and possibly its rate of growth slowed) by certain dietary factors, although the evidence in support of some of these is variable.

Myth

Prostate cancer can be prevented - or caused - by some of the things we eat.

Truth

The biggest risk factors for prostate cancer are male sex and age, over which we have no control! Although diet may affect the risk of developing the disease, the effects do not appear to be very significant.

Although there is no definite proof that factors in the diet can cause or prevent prostate cancer, there have been suggestions that certain food substances may play a role. At the moment, it seems likely that a diet low in animal fats and high in vegetables, cereals and fish may have a protective effect. As this type of diet certainly has other health benefits, such as reducing the risk of heart disease, it is worth considering.

Soy

Soy and soy products were first looked at in relation to prostate cancer because they are consumed in large quantities in Japan, which has one of the lowest incidences of the disease in the world. It seems that soy has general anti-cancer properties, possibly at least partly due to its oestrogenic effects (oestrogen can sometimes kill prostate cancer cells), although it also seems to help prevent cancers that are not hormone dependent.

Vitamin D and calcium

Although called a vitamin, vitamin D is, in fact, a steroidal hormone. Most vitamin D is synthesized in the skin by the action of sunlight, although some is also absorbed from the diet, mainly in vitamin-enriched dairy products. Its main role is in the metabolism of bone and calcium, but it has been suggested that it protects against prostate cancer by reducing the proliferation of the cancer cells. (It may also have a similar effect on colon, skin and mammary tumours.) This may help to explain why African-Americans have an increased risk of prostate cancer, as the dark pigment in their skin prevents it being able to synthesize vitamin D. Although many people believe that vitamin D has a significant role to play in the treatment of prostate cancer, the results of studies have been conflicting.

Research has shown that prostate cancer cells have receptors for vitamin D, stimulation of which inhibits the growth of the cells and triggers their death. Vitamin D may also help prevent progression of the disease.

This seems to contradict the evidence that suggests dairy products are a risk factor for prostate cancer, although the protective form of vitamin D (1,25-D) is different from the form obtained in the diet. It is also possible that the high level of calcium in dairy products suppresses the formation and circulation of 1,25-D, and studies have found a strong link between calcium intake and increased risk of prostate cancer. A high fructose intake has been shown to be associated with a lower risk of advanced prostate cancer, which may be due to its ability to boost the levels of 1,25-D.

The consistently found relationship between meat and prostate cancer could be at least partly due to the protein in meat increasing the acidity of the blood, which lowers the level of 1,25-D.

The dose of vitamin D that might be required to treat prostate cancers is not yet known. At high doses it can cause a condition called hypercalcaemia (in which there is excess calcium in the blood) and therefore synthetic forms without this effect are currently being tested.

Vitamin E

A study in Finland examining the effects of vitamin E on lung and other cancers in men who smoked showed that, although it did not seem to reduce the number of lung cancers, it did reduce prostate cancer incidence and mortality. It is possible that vitamin E inhibits the growth of the prostate cancers that are induced by a high fat intake.

Vitamin E has antioxidant properties, protecting the cell membranes from damage by substances in the body called free radicals. It has been shown in some studies to decrease cancer growth and, in high doses, may also make some parts of the immune response more effective. However, there is not yet enough evidence to show conclusively that vitamin E has a role in preventing prostate cancer.

Selenuim

Selenium is a trace element found in foods such as cereals and is essential for the action of some enzymes. Like vitamin E, it has antioxidant properties and seems to have an anti-cancer effect, although the results of trials are conflicting. In one study, men who took daily supplements of selenium over a period of several years had only about one-third the incidence of prostate cancer of men taking a placebo. Selenium also appears to be associated with a lower incidence of lung and colorectal cancers.

Lycopene

Lycopene is a carotenoid (a plant pigment found in animal tissues) and is a strong antioxidant. The main dietary source is tomatoes. Although tomato juice has been found to have little effect on the risk of developing prostate cancer, cooking tomatoes in an oil-based substance significantly increased the absorption of lycopene from the intestine. The results of one study showed that a high intake of lycopene was related to a 21% lower risk of prostate cancer. However, conflicting results have been obtained and the role of lycopene has not yet been established.

Fish oils

It has been suggested that a diet rich in fish oils can reduce the risk of prostate cancer, and research is currently underway to assess this possibility.

Complementary therapies

PC-SPES

PC-SPES is a mixture of eight different herbs that was first made by a Chinese scientist working in the USA. Studies carried out following reports by some men that it improved their prostate cancer showed it to reduce the levels of testosterone and prostate-specific antigen (PSA, see page 33) significantly and to stabilize or improve prostate cancer in some cases. Further studies are taking place to assess whether PC-SPES has a role to play in prostate cancer treatment. It is currently only available commercially and cannot be obtained on prescription from a doctor.

Up to nine capsules of PC-SPES can be taken per day, although the ideal dose is not yet known. However, it is an expensive treatment and can cause some side effects, such as breast tenderness, loss of libido, impotence, allergic reactions and blood-clotting complications.

One of the herbs included in PC-SPES is a plant form of the hormone oestrogen and it is possible that it is this component that is having the effect. (Oestrogen is known to reduce the level of PSA in some prostate cancers.)

Proslan

This is a mixture of natural ingredients (including bee pollen, vitamins and hydrangea root) that is available commercially as a treatment for both benign prostatic hyperplasia (see page 8) and prostate cancer. However, there is no clear medical evidence to show that it is effective, and one of its constituents (*Panax ginseng*) may actually increase the levels of testosterone, which stimulates the growth of some types of prostate cancer.

Saw palmetto

Extracts from the palm tree *Saw palmetto* have long been used in folk remedies for urinary problems such as difficulty in urinating and frequent passage of water at night (nocturnal polyuria, see page 15). However, although tablets, capsules or drinks made from the extracts of *Saw palmetto* have been proved to ease some of the symptoms of benign prostatic hyperplasia, there is no evidence to show that they are effective for prostate cancer.

Chapter 5

Drug trials and screening

Drug trials

It may be suggested that you take part in a clinical trial that is being run to test a new drug as a treatment for prostate cancer. These drug trials are important, as they can lead to the development of effective treatments that improve the outcome for many people with the disease. However, you are under no obligation to take part in a trial and your care will not be affected in any way if you do not wish to do so.

Clinical trials are run to decide on the most effective and safest dose of a newly developed drug, to test for any side effects it may have and to assess how effective it is in comparison (or in combination) with other available treatments.

If you do join a clinical trial, you will have frequent, comprehensive check-ups to make sure that you remain well and do not suffer any adverse effects. You should let your doctor know immediately if you have any new or worsening symptoms while taking the trial drug.

Screening

There is controversy surrounding the potential advantages of introducing screening for prostate cancer in the UK. In the USA, all men over the age of 50 are advised to be screened and the programme there has led to 200,000 new cases of prostate cancer being diagnosed each year and to an increase in radical surgery, although it is not known whether lives have been saved as a result. Screening is also routine in some other European countries. However, there are as yet no plans to set up mass screening programmes in the UK and screening is not currently available on the National Health Service (NHS). Very large trials of prostate cancer screening involving thousands of patients are currently underway in the USA and parts of Europe, the results of which should become available within the next few years.

For a screening programme to be effective, there must be a reliable and easily performed test to detect the condition and a treatment that will successfully cure it. In the view of some experts, neither of these factors currently applies to prostate cancer. Although there is a test for prostate-specific antigen (PSA, see page 33) - a protein produced by the normal prostate gland and in larger amounts in men with prostate cancer - raised levels are also sometimes present in *benign* prostate conditions.

Those who support screening point out that prostate cancer often has no symptoms in its early stages: in 20% of the approximately 20,000 new cases diagnosed in the UK each year, it has already spread beyond the prostate. Most prostate cancers are first detected during the investigation of urinary problems. However, treatment is likely to be most effective if given at an early stage of cancer development, and routine screening could therefore have a significant effect on mortality.

Those who do not support nationwide screening feel that it would not offer any benefit to the majority of men with prostate cancer but no symptoms, as the disease can have remained latent for years in elderly men, most of whom are likely to die from other causes. They therefore consider that screening would cause unnecessary anxiety and that the possible side effects of treatment, including impotence and incontinence, would not be justified.

Small-scale screening trials have been run in some parts of the UK. During a recent trial involving 5000 men, 65 were found to have prostate cancer, although none of them had any symptoms, and a further 45 had pre-cancerous changes in their prostate tissue. The usual 'pick-up' rate is about 2%, i.e. around 2 in every 100 men screened are found to have a previously undetected cancer.

The debate about screening continues, although there may be a case to be made for screening particular high-risk groups such as African Caribbean men and men with a family history of prostate cancer.

Chapter 6
Diagnosis and cancer staging investigations

Symptoms and signs

> **Symptoms** are what the patient complains of - for example pain. **Signs** are what the doctor looks for - such as a swelling.

Urinary problems can be caused by various conditions, such as kidney or bladder infections or stones, but the symptoms described below are often due to enlargement or disease of the prostate in men over the age of 50. If you experience persistent problems, you should consult your family doctor so that any necessary tests can be arranged.

❖ *Hesitancy:* urine does not flow immediately and, when it does, the flow may be slow or interrupted and not improved by straining.

❖ *Urgency:* the sudden (and possibly frequent) need to urinate associated with the feeling that you are going to wet yourself if you do not reach the toilet in time.

❖ *Frequency:* the need to urinate more often than normal.

❖ *Urge incontinence:* the sudden need to urinate, resulting in urine leaking before you reach the toilet.

❖ *Nocturia:* the need to urinate during the night, which wakes you up, although you may only pass very small amounts of urine. This symptom is distinct from nocturnal polyuria (see page 15), which involves passing large amounts of urine during the night.

You should seek medical advice if you have any other signs and symptoms such as blood in your urine (which is occasionally related to prostate problems) or are unable to urinate despite the urge to do so (which may be due to urine retention).

Myth
Prostate cancer always causes symptoms.

Truth
In many Western countries, prostate cancers are most commonly detected as a result of clinical and biochemical testing of middle-aged men - without having caused any symptoms. Even if untreated, a significant proportion of prostate cancers never cause symptoms.

Visiting your family doctor

Whether through reluctance to undergo tests and examination, a fear of what may be discovered, or an optimistic belief that the problems will go away, many men put off visiting their doctor for some time after they first experience urinary symptoms. However, it is important to seek medical advice if you have persistent and troublesome problems and, when you do so, it is helpful if you can give your doctor a note of when and how often you have been urinating and any other relevant details.

If your symptoms are not severe, your doctor may decide to monitor the situation for a while and will ask you to return for another appointment after a few weeks, or sooner if your problems get worse. For more troublesome symptoms, you may be prescribed a course of drugs or be referred to a consultant or a hospital outpatient clinic for tests.

If you develop painful, acute urine retention, you will need immediate treatment and your doctor may insert a catheter through your penis to drain the urine from your bladder (see below). You may then be sent straight to hospital for examination or an appointment may be made for you to see a urologist within a few days. (A urologist is a doctor who specializes in the urinary system and the diseases that affect it.)

> **Urinary catheters**
> Some urinary symptoms are treated by inserting a catheter to drain urine from the bladder. Local anaesthetic gel is squirted up the urethra before a lubricated catheter (a narrow, flexible tube) is carefully inserted, either through the penis and into the urethra or through a small incision made in the lower abdominal wall (a suprapubic catheter). A small balloon at the tip of the catheter is then inflated with fluid to hold it in place in the bladder. A catheter that has been inserted via the urethra has a small bag at its other end to collect the urine. If it needs to remain in place for any length of time, the bag will probably be taped to your leg and you will be shown how to empty it as it fills with urine.
>
> To remove a urinary catheter, the fluid is withdrawn from the balloon via a syringe and the tube is gently pulled out. A suprapubic catheter is removed in a similar way, and pressure is then applied to your lower abdomen by pressing on it for several minutes and leaving a pressure dressing over it for about half an hour.

Examinations and tests

If you need an examination or treatment, you may be referred to a flow clinic or urology clinic at a hospital. Before your appointment, you will probably be sent a chart on which to record how often you need to urinate and the volume of urine you pass each time. Having completed this chart over a period of several days, you should take it with you to your clinic appointment. At the clinic, tests will be done to try to discover the cause of your symptoms and the severity of any bladder obstruction. A decision will then be made about whether you need any treatment and, if you do, what type is most appropriate.

Your appointment at the flow clinic will probably last 2-3 hours and you will be told to drink plenty of fluid before or after you arrive at the hospital

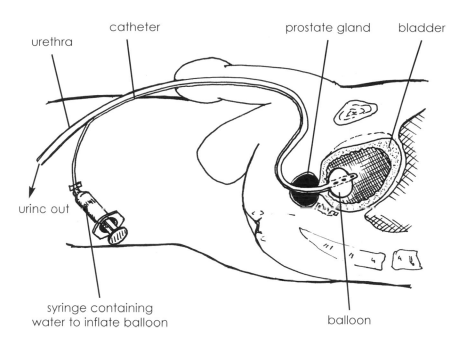

urethra　catheter　prostate gland　bladder

urine out

syringe containing
water to inflate balloon

balloon

A urinary catheter. *Once inside the bladder, the balloon is inflated with water to hold the catheter in place.*

so that your bladder is full. On arrival, you may be asked to provide a sample of urine to be checked for infection. There are several diagnostic tests that can be done and you may have some or all of them. If you are likely to need an operation, you may also have a chest X-ray to assess your general fitness for surgery.

Urine flow test

You will be asked to drink more water and, when your bladder is full again, to pass urine into a special funnel-shaped container with a meter attached to it. The meter measures and records on a chart the volume of urine you pass, its rate of flow and its pressure. A low flow rate may indicate obstruction of the bladder or urethra, and a low volume may be due to urine being retained in the bladder. This test may be repeated once or twice when you have drunk more water.

Ultrasound test

You may be given an ultrasound scan each time you have passed urine. Ultrasound (also called ultrasonography) involves passing harmless high-frequency sound waves through the body wall. When the sound waves encounter a solid object, they are reflected back like an echo and can be processed by a computer to build up an image that is displayed on a screen.

A small scanning device will be passed over your lower abdomen and any residual urine left in your bladder will be measured electronically. The procedure is completely painless.

Rectal examination

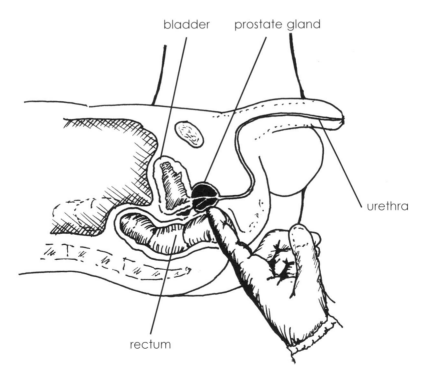

Rectal examination. *The doctor can feel the prostate gland with a gloved finger inserted through the rectum.*

As the prostate gland is close to the rectum, it can be felt during a digital rectal examination. A doctor will insert a finger into your rectum and should be able to feel whether your prostate is hard, enlarged or nodular. A large, smooth prostate indicates a benign condition, whereas a harder, nodular one may be a sign of prostate cancer. This is not a very sensitive test and, whatever its outcome, you will require further evaluation. Although digital rectal examinations are a bit uncomfortable, they are seldom painful.

Blood tests

A sample of your blood may be taken so that the levels of two substances can be measured.

Prostate-specific antigen (PSA) is a protein produced by the normal prostate. Although it is always present in the blood, its level increases with increasing age and size of the prostate and in prostatitis (see page 10). A significantly raised level of PSA may indicate the presence of prostate cancer, although the measurement has to be viewed in the context of other symptoms and signs, and further tests are always done to clarify the findings.

Myth

All men should have a PSA test to screen for prostate cancer.

Truth

There is considerable debate about screening for prostate cancer, but so far no scientifically valid study has shown it to save lives. If screening does prove to be of value, its use would be restricted to younger men, who are most likely to benefit from early diagnosis and treatment.

Intravenous urogram

Urograms provide an outline of the urinary tract. They are sometimes done to examine the kidneys if there is blood in the urine. The tests are carried out in the X-ray department and take about an hour to complete.

A simple X-ray will be taken and a contrast agent (dye) will be injected into a vein in your arm. After an hour or so, the contrast agent will start to be excreted by your kidneys and will pass through the ureters and bladder, at which time a series of X-rays will be taken. Apart from showing the size and shape of the kidneys, the X-rays will highlight any defects in your urinary system, such as stones or tumours, and may also show up any abnormalities in your bladder and, occasionally, in your prostate gland.

Further tests

If there is any doubt about the cause of your prostate problems after your visit to the flow clinic, or if cancer is suspected, you may be asked to return to have further tests.

Transrectal ultrasound scanning (TRUS)

This involves inserting an ultrasound probe into your rectum to take pictures of your prostate, which lies along the front rectal wall. You will probably be asked to lie on your left side with your knees drawn up against your chest as the ultrasound probe is inserted. The probe, which is lubricated with a jelly and covered with a condom to keep it clean, will be moved up and down within your rectum to produce two-dimensional pictures of your prostate, bladder and surrounding areas.

The scan takes about 10-15 minutes and is usually done in an investigation room in the outpatient department or day theatre area.

Prostate biopsy

A biopsy is usually done at the same time as a transrectal ultrasound scan to obtain tissue from the prostate so that a diagnosis can be made and prostate cancer can be detected or excluded.

The biopsy needle is usually inserted into the rectum and through the front part of the rectal wall into the prostate gland. Your rectal area may be cleaned with antiseptic and you may be given an antibiotic injection (and may have to take antibiotic tablets for a few days afterwards). Despite these precautions, it is still possible for infection to develop after a prostate biopsy.

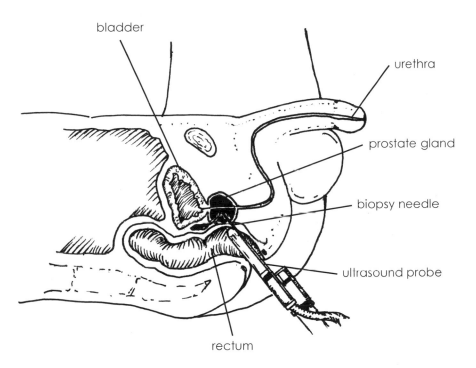

Transrectal ultrasound scanning (TRUS). *An ultrasound probe is inserted through the rectum to guide the biopsy needle into the correct position so that a small sample of tissue can be taken from the prostate gland.*

This biopsy is often done by placing a guide on an ultrasound probe and passing the biopsy needle through it. The doctor can then use the ultrasound picture to direct the procedure. The biopsy needle may be placed in a small firing device so that it can be fired in and out of your prostate gland very quickly. At least four to six samples of tissue are taken during the procedure when cancer is suspected.

Although some patients find this procedure uncomfortable, its level of discomfort does not really warrant the use of a general anaesthetic, which has its own associated risks.

The biopsy specimens will be sent to the pathology laboratory for examination and it may take 3-5 working days before the results are available. If the biopsy confirms the presence of prostate cancer, further tests such as computerized tomography (CT), magnetic resonance imaging (MRI) and isotope bone scans may be arranged for you (see below).

Because the biopsy involves cutting the tissue of the prostate gland, there may be blood in your bowel motions and urine for a day or so afterwards. As 40% of the content of semen comes from the prostate, your semen may also contain blood, possibly for several weeks.

Isotope bone scan

A bone scan may be done to detect any secondary tumours in your skeleton. A small dose of a radioactive isotope will be injected into a vein in your arm and you will be able to leave the outpatient department for 2-3 hours while waiting for it to be taken up by your bones.

When you return, you will be asked to lie on a table while a special scanning camera is passed over your body. Although the isotope is taken up by normal bone, more of it is absorbed by areas of cancer, which will show up black on the scan. The whole of your skeleton will be scanned, with particular attention being paid to your spine, pelvis and ribs. The procedure takes 30-45 minutes.

Computerized tomography (CT)

Computerized tomography is another way of producing a picture of the prostate and surrounding structures. It is done to look for regional spread of prostate cancer to the lymph nodes. You will be given an injection of a contrast agent and be asked to lie on a table, which will pass through a large hoop-shaped scanner while X-rays are taken and interpreted by a computer.

Magnetic resonance imaging (MRI)

Like CT, MRI is a form of scan that is done to detect the spread of cancer to the regional lymph nodes. The scanner in this case is a large, high-powered magnet. Following the injection of a contrast medium, you will be asked to lie on a table as it passes through a long, narrow tunnel containing the magnet. As with CT, a picture of your prostate gland and nearby structures will be produced by a computer.

It is important that you do not take anything made of metal into the scanning tunnel, because it could interfere with the magnet involved in the procedure, and you must therefore tell the doctor beforehand if you have any metal implants in your body.

Although MRI is a very useful diagnostic tool, some people are unable to tolerate it because the tunnel makes them claustrophobic.

Cancer grading and staging

There are various different systems for grading and staging cancers that are used in making the decision about what treatment is most appropriate.

Grading

Cancers can be graded according to their appearance under a microscope to give an indication of how quickly they may grow. Although there are several grading systems in use, the most common is the Gleason system, which grades prostate cancers on a scale from 1 to 5. Using this system, the arrangement of the cancer cells within the prostate is looked at and each of the two most common patterns of growth is given a score. The two scores are then added together to give a final score between 2 and 10. Low-grade cancers (grades 2-4) tend to be slow growing and less likely to spread. A high grade (8-10) means that the cancer is growing quickly and that there is a greater chance of it spreading.

Staging

Cancer staging indicates the size of the tumour and whether spread from the original site has already occurred. The primary tumour of a prostate cancer can be divided into four stages: stage 1 is a small, localized cancer, and stages 3 and 4 indicate that it has spread to other parts of the body to a lesser or greater extent. The most commonly used staging system is the TNM classification, which stages prostate cancer according to the extent of the primary tumour, whether the regional lymph nodes are involved, and whether and to what extent the cancer has spread (metastasized).

The stage at which a prostate cancer is first detected will determine which treatment is most likely to be effective. Early prostate cancers can often be cured by the surgical removal of the entire prostate gland, its capsule and the seminal vesicles, or by radiotherapy or brachytherapy (see pages 49 and 72). Locally advanced forms that have spread outside the capsule are infrequently cured and may need treatment with radiation and/or hormones. Advanced cancers with metastases at sites around the body are incurable, and palliative treatment will usually be given (i.e. treatment to reduce the impact of the symptoms, see page 67). Palliative treatments often dramatically improve the quality of a patient's life, but the duration of their effects is highly variable, ranging from a few months to many years.

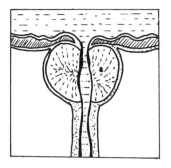

T1

Early (non-palpable) prostate cancer only detectable under the microscope

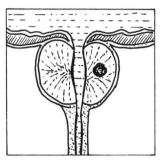

T2

Early (palpable) prostate cancer

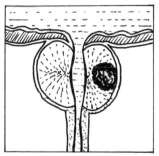

T3

Locally advanced prostate cancer - may cause urinary problems

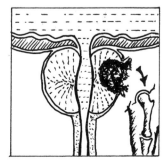

T4

Late prostate cancer - possibly with spread of cells to bone

The tumour stages of prostate cancer, T1-T4. *Staging allows an assessment to be made of how far the cancer is likely to have spread.*

Staging will involve some of the tests described above:

❖ digital rectal examination to feel the prostate gland

❖ TRUS

❖ measurement of the level of PSA in the blood, which will give a general idea of whether the cancer is localized or has spread to distant parts of the body

❖ MRI

❖ CT

❖ isotope bone scanning to look for spread to the bones.

Discussions and decisions

You will probably have an appointment with a urologist to discuss the results of your tests and the possible courses of action.

Depending on your test results and on various other factors, the urologist will discuss the possible treatment options with you. Do make sure you ask any questions you may have. Although your urologist will advise you about the best treatment for your particular condition (and may refer you to other specialists for advice), the final decision about whether to have a particular treatment is yours. You may want to ask for time to discuss things with your partner or other family members.

It is often difficult for people to take in all they are told by their doctor when they first hear they have cancer, but the hospital should have a clinical nurse specialist or nurse practitioner (or another nurse with particular experience and knowledge of urology) who you (and your partner) can ask to talk to and who will be able to give you a clear and detailed explanation of your diagnosis and any proposed treatment.

There are side effects that can occur after prostate surgery or radiotherapy and these should be explained clearly to you before you make the decision to go ahead with treatment. Some areas have patient support groups, which often provide a good opportunity for men to discuss the treatment that is being proposed for them with other men who have already undergone it. Ask your doctor for details of any groups that are available in your area.

Quality-of-life issues

On hearing that they have prostate cancer, the reaction of most people is one of shock. The diagnosis can be devastating, not only for the men directly affected, but also for their partners and families. For many people, the main consideration is whether they will be able to maintain their quality of life, which will be affected to some extent from the time they develop symptoms, throughout and beyond the period of investigations and treatment.

Apart from the physical symptoms of prostate cancer, there are psychological effects, such as fear of the unknown and of death, feelings of guilt, disbelief, anger, depression and anxiety. In addition, some people are anxious about whether they will be able to continue their normal activities, for example whether they will be able to continue to look after themselves, work, pursue their hobbies, remain mobile and maintain their social lives. It is therefore important that these quality-of-life issues are considered - by both patients and doctors - when deciding on a particular treatment.

It is now known that the quality of life of the partners of men with prostate cancer is often affected more than that of the men themselves, which is why it is essential that partners are included in the discussions between patients and their health care professionals. Family doctors, nurses, other men with prostate cancer and members of the various support groups can all play an important role: talking to other people about your concerns and worries can often help alleviate them. The groups listed in Appendix IV can offer emotional support, information and practical advice to people with prostate cancer and their friends and families, and it really is a good idea to take advantage of the help they can provide.

Chapter 7

Treatment for early prostate cancer

The type of treatment you are offered will depend to a large extent on the stage of your prostate cancer and on whether it has already spread.

Watchful waiting

In some cases, when a man has a small, slow-growing prostate cancer with mild or no symptoms, 'watchful waiting' may be recommended. This involves close and regular monitoring with blood tests, physical examinations and scans to detect any signs of progression of the disease. The basis of this 'no-treatment' option is that most men with low-grade cancer that is growing slowly and not causing any symptoms usually die of other causes before their prostate cancer becomes problematic; radical treatment might therefore cause more problems than the cancer itself. With watchful waiting, specific treatment is only given when the cancer grows and gives rise to symptoms.

Although watchful waiting has long been the standard treatment in some countries (such as Sweden), it has not been common practice in the UK or USA. However, several recent studies have shown that men with low-grade cancers confined to the prostate have an excellent prognosis without treatment, and watchful waiting has therefore now become more widely accepted.

If you are undergoing this type of observation, you should let your doctor know immediately if there is any deterioration in your condition, particularly if there are any changes in your urinary function or if you experience bone pains.

> **Myth**
> Most cases of prostate cancer don't need treatment.
>
> **Truth**
> Most prostate cancers need treatment at some point, although there is a group of less-aggressive tumours that can safely be watched and regularly assessed clinically and biochemically.

Radical prostatectomy

A small, early, localized cancer that is confined to the prostate may be treated by the removal of the entire prostate gland, its capsule and the seminal vesicles - an operation called a radical prostatectomy. Radical prostatectomy can be performed in three ways:

❖ open surgery through an incision in the abdomen

❖ open surgery through an incision in the perineum

❖ laparoscopically (see below).

All of these are major operations, which are most appropriate for the treatment of younger, fitter men. There is currently considerable debate as to whether they are justified for older men.

> **Laparoscopy**
> A laparoscopic operation involves the use of a laparoscope, a type of telescope with a video camera and light source attached. Instead of making a single large incision in the skin, the surgeon makes a series of small incisions, through which the surgical instruments and the laparoscope are inserted. A clear video picture of the operating site is then displayed on a screen in the operating theatre.

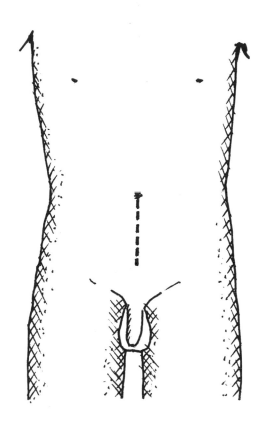

The line of the abdominal incision made for a radical prostatectomy.

Your bowel may be washed out before your operation and you will be given low-dose heparin injections and antibiotics. Although general anaesthesia is commonly used (see below), the choice of which anaesthetic you are given will depend on the type of operation you are having as well as on the normal practice of your consultant and/or hospital. You may also be given an epidural anaesthetic for pain relief (see page 48).

While you are anaesthetized, a catheter will be inserted into your bladder and the surgeon will remove your prostate gland and seminal vesicles completely. Your bladder and urethra will then be stitched together with five or six stitches over the catheter, which acts as a splint. One or two wound drains will be inserted and the wound will be closed before you are taken to the recovery room to come round from the anaesthetic.

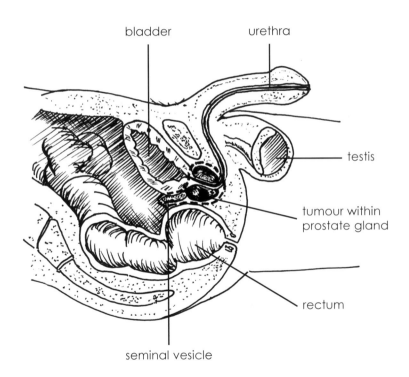

bladder

urethra

testis

tumour within prostate gland

rectum

seminal vesicle

Radical prostatectomy. *The prostate gland and seminal vesicles (encircled by the dashed line) are removed through an incision made through the abdominal wall.*

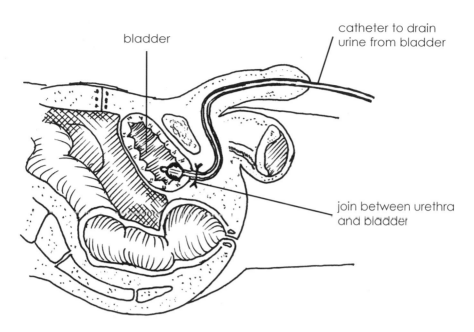

bladder

catheter to drain
urine from bladder

join between urethra
and bladder

Radical prostatectomy. *Once the prostate gland and seminal vesicles have been removed, the urethra is rejoined to the bladder and a catheter is inserted to drain urine.*

Orchidectomy

Sometimes an operation is done to remove the testes and thus reduce the body's production of the male hormone testosterone on which prostate cancer depends. This is a form of hormone therapy (see page 67), although hormone injections or tablets are now used more commonly than this form of surgery to achieve similar results. Orchidectomy may control prostate cancer at an advanced stage, but it cannot cure it.

A general anaesthetic is normally given, although local or spinal anaesthesia can be used. A single incision will probably be made across your scrotum and either your testes will be cut away completely or the bulk of their tissue will be removed and the remainder sewn back together. The incision in the scrotum will then be closed with dissolvable stitches. Wound drains are not necessary, but your scrotum is likely to be bruised for a time.

Anaesthetics

A **local anaesthetic** numbs the area around the site of injection. A sedative is sometimes given at the same time to cause drowsiness or sleep.

A **spinal anaesthetic** is injected between the vertebrae of the spine into the space around the nerves in the back. The numbness it causes in the lower body lasts for 3-5 hours.

An **epidural anaesthetic** is injected through a tube into the space around the spinal cord, close to the nerves leaving the spine. It allows drugs to be given continuously to block the conduction of pain impulses up the spinal cord and causes numbness below the waist. It provides excellent pain relief and may be continued for a few days after surgery.

A **general anaesthetic** puts you to sleep so that you have no feeling in any part of your body. It can be injected into a vein in your hand or arm or given as a gas that is inhaled through a facemask.

Pelvic node dissection

Also called lymphadenectomy, this procedure is sometimes done at the same time as prostate surgery. The lymph nodes in the pelvis are removed so that they can be examined for signs of regional spread of the cancer. If secondary tumours (metastases) are discovered in the lymph nodes, the surgeon may decide not to proceed to radical surgery, as this is unlikely to result in a cure once spread has occurred. In some hospitals, the lymph nodes are removed laparoscopically (see above) several weeks before radical surgery is scheduled so that they can be examined under a microscope and a decision can be made as to whether or not to go ahead with an operation.

There is no evidence to suggest that pelvic node dissection is itself therapeutic, but it is sometimes a useful way to stage a prostate cancer before deciding on the most suitable treatment.

If you have a pelvic node dissection at the same time as a radical prostatectomy, the lymph nodes will probably be excised first. The group of nodes that drain lymph from the prostate will be dissected out and the lymph vessels tied off. If there is any doubt about whether the lymph nodes contain malignant tissue, they will be sent immediately to the histology laboratory for examination while you are still anaesthetized. Once the laboratory results have been obtained, a decision will be made about whether or not to proceed to radical prostatectomy. If there is already cancer in your pelvic nodes, it will not be eliminated by the removal of your prostate gland and your operation may therefore be abandoned. Your surgeon should have discussed this possibility with you beforehand. When you are fully awake, the surgeon will explain the findings to you and talk about other treatment options.

Myth

If I have had an operation called transurethral resection of the prostate (TURP) to remove part of my prostate gland, I am no longer at risk of getting prostate cancer.

Truth

This is a common misconception. TURP involves making a hole in the middle of the prostate gland (similar to coring an apple) to allow someone to urinate more freely. However, there is always some prostate tissue remaining, and therefore still a risk of developing prostate cancer. Only *radical prostatectomy* removes the whole of the prostate gland.

Radiotherapy

Instead of radical surgery, radiotherapy is sometimes the primary treatment for younger men with localized prostate cancer or cancer in the very early stages of local spread. It can also help relieve the pain caused by secondary tumours in the bones, in which case it may be given at the same time as hormone therapy, or at a later date if pain subsequently recurs (see page 70). Occasionally, the treatment has to be repeated.

Some of the details given below are the same when radiotherapy is used to relieve the symptoms of bone pain in advanced disease, but specific aspects of this type of palliative treatment are dealt with on page 70.

Radiotherapy involves the use of high-energy radiation (X-rays) to destroy cancer cells. Although the X-rays damage the DNA in all cells in the targeted area, normal cells can usually repair themselves within a couple of hours, whereas the cancer cells take longer to do so and, after repeated radiation treatment, are eventually destroyed. If it is thought that the cancer may have spread to the regional pelvic lymph nodes, these may also be treated with radiotherapy.

Radiotherapy can be given:

❖ by **external beam** - the most commonly used form (described below),

❖ as **conformal radiotherapy** - which is similar to external beam but involves applying radiation to a smaller, better-targeted area,

❖ as **brachytherapy** - which involves the use of radioactive implants (see page 72).

Receiving your treatment

Radiotherapy as a primary treatment is usually given in several separate sessions (for example every weekday for 6 weeks or more), each lasting only a few minutes. Before the treatment starts, a total radiation dose is calculated and divided into several smaller amounts to be given at each treatment session. Although different treatment centres may divide the total dose differently, the outcome is generally the same.

If you are going to have radiotherapy, you may be sent an appointment for pre-treatment planning so that your doctor can decide how best to

> **Radiologists** are doctors who have been trained to interpret X-rays and to administer the dyes etc. that are used for some types of X-ray examination.
>
> **Radiographers** are technicians who have undergone a 3-year degree course and are qualified to operate X-ray machinery and to administer radiation treatment under the guidance of a doctor.
>
> **Radiotherapists** (or **radiation oncologists**) are doctors who specialize in the treatment of cancer using radiation. Most also administer other types of cancer treatment, such as chemotherapy.
>
> **Oncologists** are physicians who have specialist training in all aspects of cancer, particularly radiotherapy and chemotherapy, but not surgery.

administer it. The doctor in charge of your treatment may be a clinical oncologist or a radiotherapist (see above). During the pre-treatment planning or on your first visit for radiotherapy, a radiographer will explain the procedures to you. Do ask any questions, however trivial they may seem, and do not be afraid to ask for something to be explained again if you have not understood it. If you are at all worried as your treatment progresses, talk to the radiographer on a subsequent visit.

When you enter the treatment room for your first radiotherapy session, you will be asked to lie on a couch and the doctor will mark the area to be treated by drawing around it on your skin using a felt-tip pen. The X-ray machine will be lowered until it almost touches your abdomen and you will be told to keep very still while your treatment is in progress.

Once the machine has been set up, all the medical staff will leave the treatment room to protect themselves against repeated exposure to radiation. A radiographer will watch you closely through a window or on a

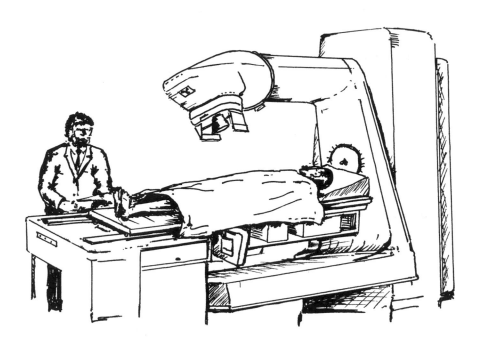

External beam radiotherapy. *Radiation is targeted on the prostate gland and surrounding tissues to destroy the cancer cells.*

television monitor. If you are concerned or require any assistance, simply raise your hand and the process will be stopped immediately. There will also be an intercom system so the radiographer can hear and speak to you. The treatment only lasts a couple of minutes.

Side effects

Some men experience side effects, which usually stop when their treatment finishes. Others suffer no ill-effects and are able to continue their normal activities between treatment sessions. If you do feel tired during and immediately after your course of treatment, it may be a good idea to arrange to work part-time for a while so that you can rest when you need to.

Diarrhoea, cystitis-like problems and the passage of blood in the urine and faeces are common during radiotherapy because parts of the bowel and the bladder are included in the treatment area. However, the side effects can be quite severe and a small number of men are left with more permanent problems. You should tell the radiographer or a doctor if you do experience any side effects, as there are medicines you can take to help relieve diarrhoea and ways to manage frequent urination.

You will lose the hair within the treated area, but it will grow again once your treatment stops.

There is a 30-40% risk of impotence following radical radiotherapy and this possibility should be explained and discussed with you before your treatment starts.

Hostel wards

Some hospitals have hostel wards, which are usually open from Monday to Friday for use by people who would have to travel some distance each day for their treatment. These wards provide a bed and meals. They are suitable for people who are able to look after themselves and are therefore ideal for those undergoing daily radiotherapy treatment who are otherwise in good health.

If you think it might be helpful for you to stay in a hostel ward, ask your doctor about this before your treatment starts.

Chapter 8

After your operation

In hospital

If you have had a radical prostatectomy performed through an incision in your abdomen, you are likely to have some abdominal pain and may not be able to eat for a day or two until you have gradually built up your fluid intake. If your operation was done through the perineum or laparoscopically, you will probably be able to eat immediately after it.

When you wake up from the anaesthetic, you will have a urinary catheter, one or two wound drains and an intravenous drip, through which you will be given specially balanced fluids to replace the fluid you lost during your operation. You may also have a nasogastric tube to drain your stomach.

As well as draining the urine from your bladder, the urinary catheter also acts as a splint to support the join between your bladder and urethra as it heals. A close check will be kept on your fluid balance while you are in hospital to make sure the amount of urine you are passing relates to the amount of fluid you are taking in. Therefore it is important that you always ask a nurse to empty your catheter bag rather than doing it yourself.

After a couple of days, when there is less blood and fluid leaking from your abdominal wound, the wound drain(s) will be taken out. You may be given pain relief intravenously, by epidural (see page 48) or using a patient-controlled analgesia machine (see page 55), and will continue to be given low-dose heparin injections until you are mobile (see page 61).

The intravenous drip will be taken down when you are able to drink again and your fluid intake will gradually be increased over a couple of days, until are eating a light and then a normal diet. You should try to drink up to 3 litres of fluid a day to help flush out your bladder, gradually reducing to about 1.5 litres a day.

Patient-controlled analgesia

If you are given one of these machines, you will be able to control the amount of pain-killing drugs (analgesics) you receive.

The machine is basically a pump, which provides your body with a predetermined amount of drug each time you press a button. The drug is usually delivered via a cannula inserted into a vein in the hand or arm or directly into the skin on the lower abdomen. The machine is programmed so that you cannot receive more than a safe level of the drug. When you press the button, your pain should start to reduce within 5-10 minutes. If it does not do so, you can press the button again - as often as you like.

Because the safety device that prevents you receiving too much of the drug will have been programmed specifically for you, it is important that you do not let anyone else use your machine.

If your pain is not relieved despite pressing the button several times, tell a nurse or doctor so that the machine can be reset to give you a stronger dose of the drug, if appropriate.

There is a counter on the machine that will indicate how many times you have pressed the button and how much of the drug you have received. A nurse or doctor will check this counter daily and reset it to give you a lower dose when your pain starts to improve.

You are unlikely to need to use a patient-controlled analgesia machine for more than 24-48 hours, after which you can take analgesic tablets.

Leaving hospital

You will probably be able to leave hospital within 5-7 days, still with a urinary catheter in place, or possibly sooner than this if you have had a laparoscopic or perineal operation. You should not drive for at least a couple of weeks - preferably not for 4-6 weeks. If necessary, you may be able to make use of hospital transport to take you home, but if you think you may need it, you should tell a nurse some time before you are due to leave hospital, to allow time for the necessary arrangements to be made.

When you leave hospital, you may be given a letter to deliver to your doctor's surgery as soon as possible, although it may be sent by post from the hospital. This letter is important, as it will let your family doctor know the details of your operation and of any further treatment you may need.

At home

Once you are at home, you will have to take things easy for a while. People recover from surgery at different rates, but it may be several weeks or more until you feel any real benefit, and some men do not feel they have made a full recovery for up to 6 months.

Returning to normal activity

You may feel tired and a bit depressed for anything from a few days to a few weeks. This is quite normal and will eventually pass. However, if you continue to feel depressed, you should talk to your doctor, as you may need counselling and/or short-term drug treatment to help you get over it. For the first couple of weeks at least, you should go on only short walks (less than a mile) and avoid driving and any strenuous activity. Playing golf, cycling and similar sports should not be resumed for about 3 months after your operation. Always ask your doctor if you are in any doubt about something you want to do.

Sex

You should not have sexual intercourse for about 6 weeks after your operation, by which time your internal wound will have had a chance to heal.

Fluid intake and urine output

You should continue to drink plenty - about 2 litres a day for the first week you are at home and then as much as possible. You may continue to have some leakage of urine and may need to urinate frequently and during the night, but these problems will gradually resolve. Avoiding drinking too much just before you go to bed may help reduce the number of times you have to get up in the night. You can wear a small pad (available from any pharmacy) inside your underpants if urine leaks when you laugh or cough. If you continue to have continence problems, ask at your doctor's surgery to see a district nurse or for a referral to a nurse specialist for advice.

You may pass a small amount of blood through your urethra when you have a bowel motion, but this is normal and nothing to worry about.

Constipation

Constipation can be a problem in the first few days after surgery and you may be given suppositories while you are in hospital. Once you are at home, you should avoid becoming constipated because straining may cause your internal wound to bleed. You may need to take laxatives if a high-fibre diet does not help. Ask your doctor for advice if the problem persists.

Returning to work

Unless you have a heavy manual job, you will probably be able to return to work about 2-3 months following a radical prostatectomy. If you are in any doubt, ask your doctor for advice and for a certificate to enable you to stay off work, which can be renewed on request.

Follow-up appointments

You will probably be given an appointment to see your consultant about 2 weeks after your operation so that your progress can be checked, and a cystogram may be done (see below).

> A **cystogram** involves squirting a dye down the side of the urinary catheter and taking a series of X-rays. The dye will leak out through (and reveal) any gaps in the join between your bladder and urethra. If healing is complete, the catheter can be removed; if not, it will have to remain in place for a further week or two.

A blood test will be done to measure your level of prostate-specific antigen (PSA, see page 33). If your prostate gland and the cancer have been removed completely, your PSA level should have returned to normal. If all is well, you may be seen again after a further 3 months and possibly 6 monthly thereafter to check your PSA level and make sure any incontinence or impotence is improving. The intervals between your check-ups will depend on the normal practice of your consultant. If you have advanced prostate cancer, you are likely to be seen every 3-6 months.

When you go for your follow-up appointments, you may find it helpful to take with you a note of any questions you have so that you can make sure you remember to ask them.

Exercises

Once the urinary catheter has been taken out, you can start doing pelvic-floor exercises to help you regain control of your bladder. It is a good idea to practise doing these exercises before your operation so that you get used to them.

If you had to strain to pass urine before your operation, it will be a few days before the muscles of your bladder return to a relaxed state. Once the urinary catheter has been removed, you can do some simple exercises to tighten the perineal muscles around your urethra and to help prevent urine leakage. The more often you do these exercises, the sooner you will regain bladder control.

Exercise 1
Every time you urinate, tighten your perineal muscles by trying to stop the flow of urine midstream for a few seconds

Exercise 2
Standing upright, pull in your stomach muscles, count to 10 and then relax. Do this exercise each time you stand up and at least every hour to gain maximum effect.

Exercise 3
While standing, sitting or lying down, tighten the muscles of your anus by pulling them up as though you were trying to stop a bowel motion. Do this exercise about every 10 minutes, while breathing normally.

Chapter 9

Possible complications of surgery

All operations carry a small risk of general complications such as deep vein thrombosis or chest infection, but there are also other potential complications that are specifically related to prostate surgery. Although minor post-operative problems are fairly common, serious ones are rare. However, it is important to be aware of what could go wrong so that you know when to seek medical advice.

General complications

The following are the complications that can occur after any type of surgery and the minor side effects associated with the use of general anaesthesia, which should only last a day or two.

Sore throat

You may have a sore throat for a couple of days after a general anaesthetic. This is due to the 'dry' anaesthetic gases or to a tube being put down your throat to help you breathe.

Muscle aches

The muscle relaxants used during anaesthesia can cause muscle aches and pains, but these should clear up within about 48 hours.

Chest infection

Chest infection is possible following general anaesthesia for any type of operation and is particularly common in smokers. Deep breathing is important post-operatively to keep the lungs clear and, if necessary, a physiotherapist will visit you on the hospital ward to advise you about appropriate exercises.

Pyrexia

Pyrexia is fever. It can occur in the first 24 hours after surgery, but if it persists, its cause will have to be investigated. It may be due to a chest or wound infection or to deep vein thrombosis, although after prostate surgery it is most likely to indicate a urinary tract infection. Urinary infection can occasionally result in bacteraemia (a condition caused by bacteria in the circulating blood) or septicaemia (a more severe infection involving the invasion of the blood by large numbers of bacteria that spread throughout the body). Antibiotics are given for at least a few days after surgery to reduce these risks.

Deep vein thrombosis

Deep vein thrombosis occurs when blood clots form in the deep veins of the body - usually in the calf veins of the legs. Its potential danger is associated with the risk of the blood clot breaking away and lodging in an organ such as the lungs, where it causes what is known as a pulmonary embolism, with possibly fatal results.

While you are in hospital, you will be given special anti-embolism stockings to wear and a course of low-dose heparin injections to help prevent a thrombosis developing. Thromboses usually cause inflammation of the surrounding area (making the skin red and hot to the touch) and possibly pain or an aching feeling. It you do develop a thrombosis, it is important that you receive treatment with a course of higher-dose heparin or warfarin to break up the clot and avoid more serious complications.

Complications after radical prostatectomy

There is inevitably a wider range of complications that can occur after invasive surgery and you should let your doctor know if there is anything you are concerned about.

Pain

Although it is normal to have some pain in the abdominal wound after a prostatectomy, it is unusual for it to be severe. Severe, persistent pain may be a sign that an infection is developing, which will require medical attention (see page 63).

Bleeding and bruising

There is often oozing of blood or fluid from the abdominal wound, but this is unlikely to be heavy. If it continues, and particularly if leakage occurs through the wound dressing and soils your clothes, medical advice should be sought. On rare occasions, a second operation is required to tie off or cauterize a bleeding blood vessel that has been overlooked or that has started to bleed again post-operatively.

Occasionally, blood that does not escape through the edges of the wound may cause severe bruising, which sometimes only develops several days after surgery. Although the sight of the bruise may be distressing, treatment to release the blood that has accumulated under the skin is only rarely necessary.

Haematoma

In rare cases, after any type of surgery, a haematoma may develop. A haematoma is a swelling that is full of blood and is caused by a blood vessel continuing to bleed or re-opening after surgery. It can sometimes result from a disturbance of the normal blood-clotting mechanisms of the body, for example due to anticoagulants such as heparin. There are also inherited bleeding disorders, such as haemophilia, which cause a similar disturbance of the blood-clotting mechanism, but these conditions will be taken into account before any operation is considered.

Haematoma development is accompanied by pain, the formation of a hard swelling and possibly a reddish purple discoloration of the skin. Bruising may appear around the wound or at some distance from it over the next few days. Your may develop a fever and high body temperature if the wound becomes infected.

If you think a haematoma is forming (or has formed) once you have left hospital, you should contact your family doctor or consultant for advice. The blood is likely to be re-absorbed spontaneously within 3-4 weeks without the need for any treatment, but if heavy bleeding continues, with increased pain and swelling, you may need surgery to close off the blood vessel that is causing it. Your doctor may also advise you to have specialized blood tests to check that your blood-clotting factors are normal.

Wound infection

Infection can sometimes occur in the abdominal wound following a prostatectomy and is indicated by pain, swelling, heat and redness, possibly with leakage of pus or infected fluid and a high body temperature. As most modern wound dressings are transparent, it is now much easier to examine wounds for signs of infection.

If an infection develops, the wound may just need to be cleansed or it may require treatment with antibiotics. Occasionally, some of the stitches (which provide potential sites for the concentration of germs) may have to be removed to allow an infected discharge to escape. You should seek medical attention if you have any signs of an infection.

Very occasionally, possibly weeks or months after surgery, an infection can develop when foreign bodies such as suture material have been left within the wound.

Nerve damage

The small nerves supplying the skin over the lower abdomen are usually damaged when an incision is made during surgery, which can occasionally cause a small area around the wound to remain permanently numb. Although the size of the affected area will decrease with time, the sensation may never return completely.

Very rarely, small, painful, tender areas form in part of the scar, which may be due to a swelling of the cut nerve endings known as a neuroma. Nerve damage can cause pain in the wound, which will be relieved temporarily by the injection of local anaesthetic. Continued pain may respond to steroid injection. Only rarely is surgery needed to remove a painful nodule.

Constipation

Constipation is not uncommon in the first few days after a prostatectomy. You may be given laxative suppositories while in hospital to prevent you having to strain to empty your bowel. You should have a high-fibre diet once you are at home, but if constipation persists, ask your doctor about taking a laxative.

Difficulty in passing urine

Passing urine may be difficult for several days after the catheter has been removed following a radical prostatectomy, sometimes due to pain. If urine retention occurs, a catheter may have to be left in place longer than normal to empty the bladder until you are able to urinate spontaneously (see page 30). Always seek medical advice if you appear to be retaining urine.

Stenosis

Occasionally, urine comes out in a spray or narrow stream after surgery due to constriction (called stenosis or stricture) of the neck of the bladder. If necessary, this can be corrected by a small operation to dilate the bladder neck.

Incontinence

Temporary incontinence is relatively common after radical prostate surgery and may persist for weeks or even months.

If leakage of urine occurs post-operatively as a result of the bladder being damaged during the operation, a catheter may be left in place until the bladder has healed.

It is also possible for the operation itself to affect the sphincter that closes off the flow of urine from the bladder. This is usually a temporary problem, which will improve with time.

However, some 3-5% of prostate operations result in permanent incontinence, which may require an operation to insert an artificial urinary sphincter.

Sterility

Because semen is no longer produced after radical prostatectomy, men who have had this operation become sterile.

Loss of libido

Occasionally, men experience a loss of interest in sex after their prostate gland has been removed, and this is a possibility you should consider and discuss with your doctor before your operation. Although this loss of libido can be a cause of concern for some men, the risk must be weighed against the potential benefits of a radical prostatectomy for someone with prostate cancer.

Impotence

Impotence is relatively common following radical prostate surgery, and is something you should discuss with your surgeon before your operation. Some surgeons use an intra-operative nerve stimulator (called the Cavermap) to try to identify the erectile nerves during radical prostatectomy so that they can avoid injuring them. You may want to ask whether your surgeon uses this technique - or at least enquire about the potency results of your particular surgeon after this type of operation.

Other sexual effects

A significant proportion of men experience a change in their sensation of orgasm after a prostatectomy, which for some reduces their enjoyment of sex.

Risks of general anaesthesia

The use of a general anaesthetic always involves a certain risk, although the advances that have been made in anaesthesia over recent years have been tremendous. However, complications still sometimes occur and, on very rare occasions, people die during operations. Therefore, the small but real risks need to be understood and considered.

If the supply of oxygen to the brain is interrupted during anaesthesia, there are two possible outcomes: death may occur without the patient ever waking up, or the patient may wake brain damaged and possibly paralysed. It should be emphasized, however, that these risks are small, and both the surgeon and the anaesthetist will have given careful consideration to your general state of health and all other relevant factors before deciding to go ahead with your operation and anaesthesia.

Chapter 10

Treatment of advanced prostate cancer

Radiotherapy or hormone therapy may slow the growth of an advanced prostate cancer or help relieve its symptoms. These treatments, which can sometimes prevent the cancer from growing for many months or years but which cannot cure it, are called palliative. Chemotherapy is rarely used to treat prostate cancer. Although it is sometimes a palliative treatment for some types of metastatic cancer (i.e. cancer that has spread to other parts of the body), it is relatively ineffective for prostate cancer.

For people with incurable cancer, there is now a wide range of care and support available from hospices as well as specially trained nurses based in hospitals, cancer centres and the community, and there is a great deal that can be done to make living with cancer a less frightening and stressful experience for sufferers and their families. Palliative care is not just for people who are about to die; it is long-term care that can continue for months or years, and many people take advantage of the support that is available to improve their quality of life.

In Britain, hospice-based care and the support of Macmillan nurses (see page 76) are free to all who need them and are funded by charities or by the National Health Service.

Hormone therapy

Hormone therapy blocks the actions of the male hormones (androgens) produced by the body that affect the growth and function of prostate tissue. It can be used to shrink a prostate cancer or to slow its rate of growth by removing the male hormone on which its cells depend. However, there is no firm evidence that early hormone treatment improves the survival of men with prostate cancer. Some 60-70% of men who already have metastatic disease in the bones when hormone treatment is started respond well, 10-20% respond reasonably and 10-20% show no response.

There are various types of hormone therapy, although they probably all have similar (if not identical) clinical effects.

Bilateral orchidectomy

The main male hormone involved in prostate cancer is testosterone, which is produced by the testes. Although bilateral orchidectomy is a surgical procedure to remove both testes (see page 47), it is strictly a hormone treatment in that it results in the loss of the main source of testosterone.

LHRH analogues

Testosterone is under the control of another hormone called luteinizing hormone (LH), which is produced by the pituitary gland in the brain. LH is in turn controlled by luteinizing hormone-releasing hormone (LHRH), which is produced in the hypothalamus in the brain. Various artificial forms of LHRH (called LHRH analogues) have been developed to treat prostate cancer. If given continuously, these 'turn off' the pituitary gland and stop it producing LH, thus halting the production of testosterone.

The LHRH analogues are usually given as injections, either once a month or once every 3 months. The most commonly used forms in the UK are goserelin (Zoladex) and leuprorelin (Prostap). Another example is triptorelin (De-capeptyl). Zoladex is a pellet that is injected under the skin of the abdominal wall. Prostap is a powder that is dissolved and injected just under the skin or muscle. You may be given your first injection by your consultant, or possibly a radiotherapist or oncologist, but are likely to be given subsequent injections at your local health centre.

There is an initial complication associated with the use of the LHRH analogues, in that they tend to turn the regulatory system of the pituitary up for a couple of weeks, thus increasing the levels of hormone produced in the body. This effect is reduced by giving the drugs in combination with an anti-androgen drug (e.g. cyproterone acetate - see below) for the first couple of weeks until the hormone system has turned itself off.

Anti-androgens

The anti-androgens are a group of drugs that block the effects of the male hormones (the androgens) on the prostate cells. They are used to treat prostate cancer either alone or in combination with LHRH analogues (see 'Maximal androgen blockade', below). They include flutamide (Drogenil), bicalutamide (Casodex) and cyproterone acetate (Cyprostat) and are given as tablets, sometimes for many years.

Anti-androgens are not usually used as the main hormonal therapy for men with prostate cancer, but may be of value in younger men because they reduce osteoporosis and impotence, which are common consequences of bilateral orchidectomy and of long-term LHRH analogue therapy. They appear to be as effective as the LHRH analogues, but some people may find the need to take daily tablets less convenient than having monthly or 3-monthly injections. Flutamide and bicalutamide can cause breast pain, breast enlargement and gastrointestinal problems; cyproterone acetate can cause shortness of breath and tiredness.

Maximal androgen blockade

Maximal androgen blockade (MAB) is a type of hormone therapy that combines orchidectomy or the use of LHRH analogues with anti-androgens. The aim of MAB is to prevent the androgens that are synthesized by the adrenal glands from stimulating the growth of prostate cancers. It has been suggested that this treatment may slightly improve survival for younger men (in their fifties and sixties) with advanced disease. However, because of its side effects, MAB is not widely used in Britain at the present time.

Oestrogens

In the past, a group of female hormones called oestrogens were used to treat advanced prostate cancer. Although these were effective in controlling the cancer, they caused more side effects than the other treatments mentioned here. At high doses, they tend to cause feminization, including enlargement of the breasts and breast pain, and increase the risk of heart disease when taken in the long term. They are therefore not now used routinely, although several trials are currently examining the role of low-dose oestrogens.

Radiotherapy

Apart from its use as a cure for localized prostate cancer in younger men (see Chapter 7), radiotherapy can be a useful treatment to relieve bone pain in men with advanced disease. It may be given at the same time as hormone therapy, or at a later date if the hormone therapy stops working. A single treatment of the affected area is sometimes enough to relieve bone pain, but it will take 7-10 days for its effects to become fully apparent. Alternatively, the radiation dose can be divided into fractions that are given during several treatment sessions over a week or two.

For severe bone pain due to metastases, a single high dose of radiation may be given to half the body (called hemi-body radiotherapy). Alternatively, a radioactive liquid (strontium-89) may be injected into a vein, from where it is taken up by the areas of bone affected by the cancer. This treatment does not become fully effective for about 3-4 weeks. It has no major side effects and, if it successfully relieves the bone pain, it can be repeated after 3-4 months. However, it has not become a widely available treatment in Britain.

Advanced prostate cancer can affect the bones of the spine, which may put pressure on the nerves of the spinal cord. This is a serious condition, which can lead to permanent paralysis unless it is treated promptly with radiotherapy. Therefore, if you develop weakness of your arms or legs or numbness of your skin, you should report these symptoms to your doctor immediately.

Chapter 11

Newer treatments

Recent advances in our understanding of the biology of cancer cells have led to the research that is currently being done to try to find a safe and effective treatment for prostate cancer. However, although improvements have been made in the treatment of localized disease (see below), there are, as yet, no effective therapies for metastatic, hormone-independent prostate cancer, which has a relatively poor prognosis.

New drugs

Several clinical trials are taking place to test a number of new drugs, most of which act by blocking certain signalling events within cells that enable the cancer cells to survive. It is hoped that these new drugs will prove safer than the less specific cytotoxic drugs that have been used to date.

Some of the newer drugs you may come across include:

❖ endothelin antagonists, which prevent tumours from growing new blood vessels,

❖ cyclo-oxygenase-2 (COX-2) inhibitors, which have functions similar to aspirin,

❖ osteoclast inhibitors, which affect bone metabolism,

❖ growth-factor antagonists, which block the stimulatory effects of growth factors on cancer cells.

Specific vaccines have also been produced to treat prostate cancers that are hormone independent. These act by stimulating the patient's own immune system to destroy the cancer cells and have shown promising results in a number of cases.

Several research studies are also in progress to explore the use of high-intensity ultrasound and radiofrequency energy to treat localized prostate cancer, although there is currently little evidence to support their use.

Brachytherapy

Brachytherapy is a type of radiotherapy used for the treatment of early, localized prostate cancer. It is not yet widely available in Britain. It involves the insertion of radioactive implants into the prostate gland and can be done in two ways.

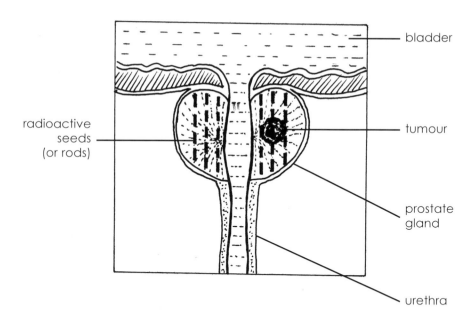

Brachytherapy. *Seeds or rods of radioactive material are inserted into the prostate gland and gradually destroy the cancer. Rods have to be removed at a later date, but the seeds can be left in place and will lose their radioactivity over a period of time.*

High-dose brachytherapy

You will be given a spinal or epidural anaesthetic before radioactive rods are implanted into your prostate gland through the skin in the area between your scrotum and anus (the perineum). During the couple of days you are in hospital, you will undergo four sessions of treatment, after which all the rods will be removed. You will be given a urinary catheter (see page 30), which will probably be taken out after a couple of weeks.

Permanent seed brachytherapy

This treatment involves the use of seeds of radioactive material, rather than rods. You will be given an ultrasound scan (see page 32) about 6 weeks before your treatment so that the exact location of the cancer can be pinpointed. Needles will be inserted through the perineal skin and into your prostate gland. This procedure is done only once, using general or spinal anaesthesia, and you will be able to leave the hospital as soon as you have recovered from the anaesthetic. The seeds remain in your body, gradually losing their radioactivity, but will not cause any harm to people who touch or come close to you.

There is currently only limited evidence concerning the effectiveness of brachytherapy compared to radical surgery and external beam radiotherapy.

Cryotherapy

This treatment (which is also called cryosurgery) uses liquid nitrogen to freeze the tissue of a tumour at a temperature of -50°C or lower, which kills the prostate cells. The liquid nitrogen is contained within an instrument called a cryoprobe, which is pushed into the cancer or placed against it. The cryoprobe will be inserted through your rectum, and ultrasound scans (see page 32) will be used to guide it into place. You may receive a course of repeated freezing and thawing.

Cryotherapy is not widely available and is only used in the treatment of smaller cancers that have not extended beyond the capsule around the prostate gland. It is not yet known how effective it is in the long term, but it has been used when prostate cancer has returned after radiotherapy. However, as it is still being experimentally assessed, it is not a routine treatment, although it may become so in the future.

The side effects of cryosurgery include bleeding and infection in the prostate gland and possibly temporary incontinence and impotence.

Chapter 12

Hospice care

Your family doctor, consultant or specialist cancer nurse may suggest you consider involving a hospice in your care if you have metastatic prostate cancer. Many people are shocked at this suggestion, because they imagine hospices to be places to go to die. However, although some people do choose to spend their last days in a hospice, their main role is to support cancer patients - and their families - and to help them remain well and to live as full and normal a life as possible for as long as possible, which in many cases means continuing support for years. Hospice staff work with family doctors to plan the best care for their patients.

Hospices have several aims:

❖ to help cancer patients live full and happy lives

❖ to provide pain relief and to control any other symptoms of cancer that may arise

❖ to counsel and support cancer patients and their families

❖ to offer advice and information about the grants and financial assistance that may be available

❖ to provide regular home visits to support and care for cancer patients and their families and to enable people to be cared for in their own homes rather than in hospitals

❖ to provide education and courses on palliative care for nurses and doctors.

Some hospices also have in-patient facilities where people can go if they have symptoms that need to be brought under control, or simply to give their carers at home a week or two's respite. Many also have day-care facilities where cancer sufferers can spend the day involved in leisure activities such as painting, woodwork or making jewellery, and where they can have their hair cut, be bathed if this is becoming difficult at home, talk to a doctor or social worker, or just sit and chat in a friendly and supportive environment.

Specialist nurses based within hospices or in the community work closely with family doctors - who remain in overall charge of their patients' care - as well as with community nurses and social workers. Their special skills and experience enable them to co-ordinate the care their patients receive and to make sure they have the emotional support and medical treatment they need.

Some people prefer not to be referred to a hospice, and some manage well alone, but many who do accept this help find their quality of life and ability to cope with their disease much improved.

Macmillan nurses

Macmillan Cancer Relief was set up in the UK in 1911 to provide care and support for cancer patients. This national charity now helps to improve the quality of life for cancer patients and their families at home, in hospitals and in special cancer units.

The charity has trained more than 2000 Macmillan nurses - all with at least 5 years' experience - who work in the community and in hospitals around Britain. It continues to fund these specially trained nurses for up to 3 years in posts in hospitals, after which the health authority takes over the financial responsibility.

Your family doctor or district nurse may suggest involving a Macmillan nurse to help with your care. Macmillan nurses play a similar role to that of hospice-based nurses, giving advice and emotional support to patients and their families and working closely with other medical professionals to advise about pain relief and symptom control. They are also involved in training doctors and nurses to help them develop the special skills required for the care of cancer patients and, with hospice staff, have been largely responsible for the increased awareness of other health professionals to the particular care these patients need.

Other treatment centres

The effects of complementary or alternative therapies are difficult to assess, in part because they are often only resorted to by people for whom conventional medicine has no more to offer in terms of cure.

There are a few private centres in the UK that advocate special, non-medical therapies to help people 'fight' or live with cancer. Your family doctor, consultant or a specialist nurse should be able to give you details of any such centres in your area, and the associations listed in Appendix IV will also have this information. Although, in the UK, the NHS does not fund alternative therapy centres, some have trust funds to help meet the costs for those who cannot afford them.

Appendix I

Different types of treatment

Treatment	Operation required	Stage of disease treated	What is involved	Potential for cure
Watchful waiting	No	Early	Regular monitoring	No - but suitable for 'low-risk' tumours
Radical prostatectomy	Yes - surgery can be done via several routes	Early	Major operation to remove prostate gland	May cure cancer completely
Orchidectomy	Yes	Late	Operation to remove testes	No - but may control disease and improve survival
External beam radiation	No	Early and late	X-ray treatment	Yes
Brachytherapy	No, but is done using X-ray guidance	Early	Radioactive seeds implanted into prostate (an invasive procedure)	Still being evaluated
Hormone therapy	No	Late	Tablets/injections/ implants	No - but may control disease and improve survival

continued:-

Side effects	Other negative aspects	Positive aspects
None	Patient may find uncertainty worrying Risk of disease progression Treatment may be required eventually	Can continue normal life
Risk of impotence (up to 70%) Risk of some degree of incontinence (5-15%) Infertility	Will not cure metastases Involves up to 1 week in hospital and 4-6 weeks off work Small risk from general anaesthetic	Reassurance of cure - depending on findings during surgery
Possible psychological problems Decreased libido	Additional treatment may be required	A 'one-off' procedure Hormone injections not required
May affect function of bladder and rectum May cause short-term diarrhoea/cystitis Risk of impotence (up to 30%)	Daily treatment required for 6 weeks Likely to be accompanied by some form of hormone treatment	Non-invasive out-patient procedure No anaesthetic required
Few If prostate is already enlarged and obstructing bladder, can increase the urinary symptoms	Not widely available in the UK Can cause worsening of bladder symptoms Not given if TURP done previously	No stay in hospital necessary Short recovery period, only 1 or 2 days off work
May cause hot flushes May cause breast enlargement/tenderness Decreased libido	Effectiveness may wear off in time	Treatment can be stopped if severe side effects are experienced Can be given intermittently Can be self-administered

Appendix II

Questions and answers

1. I have been told I have prostate cancer and am due to start radiotherapy next month. Will this treatment cure my cancer and is it safe to delay starting it this long?

If the cancer is still localized, there is a good chance that radiotherapy will cure it. Prostate cancers are usually slow growing and progress over a matter of years, so there should be no reason why delaying your treatment for a few weeks will affect your chances of cure. Do talk to your doctor, or ask for an appointment with a nurse specialist at your hospital so that you can raise any questions you have and your condition and the proposed treatment can be explained to you.

2. I have heard that prostate surgery makes men impotent. I am 63 and have been advised that I need a radical prostatectomy, but I do not want to have this operation if this is the case. Is there an alternative treatment with less drastic effects?

There is a risk of impotence following radical prostatectomy, which has been estimated to be up to 70%. Your urology consultant will be able to give you more details about this and you should ask your family doctor to make an appointment for you, or ring your consultant's secretary. Alternatively, you could ask to talk to a nurse specialist at your hospital to discuss why this particular treatment has been chosen for you and to go over things in more detail. Although the final decision about whether or not to undergo surgery is yours, do bear in mind that your doctor probably feels this offers the best chance of curing your prostate cancer and that its benefits are outweighed by the risk of impotence.

3. I am due to have a prostate operation that I understand will involve open surgery and quite a long scar. A friend who had a similar operation doesn't seem to have any scar at all. Should I find another surgeon who can do it the same way?

Although most prostate operations for benign conditions are now done through the urethra by inserting instruments into the penis, open prostate surgery is necessary to remove the prostate gland altogether to treat prostate cancer. It sounds as though an open operation *is* needed in your case, but do ask your family doctor or consultant why this type of surgery has been chosen for you.

4. My father is 74 and has various urinary problems that have recently been diagnosed as due to prostate cancer. His doctor has suggested 'watchful waiting', but surely my father needs urgent treatment now to get rid of the cancer before it spreads?

Your father's doctor may feel that an operation is not necessary at the present time if the cancer is small and not aggressive and the symptoms are not severe. If your father's general health is poor and the cancer is likely to grow so slowly that it will not cause any serious problems during his lifetime, the risks of surgery may be thought to be greater than those posed by the cancer itself. If the cancer has already spread to other parts of your father's body, removal of the prostate gland will not cure it, but watchful waiting will enable any further symptoms to be dealt with as they arise.

Your father's situation will be monitored regularly and action will be taken as and when it becomes necessary. Your father should let his doctor know immediately if he detects any change in his symptoms. Do ask to talk to your father's doctor yourself if you are concerned.

5. I have been diagnosed as having prostate cancer. What are the chances of it spreading?

Any cancer will eventually spread to other parts of the body, but the majority of prostate cancers are relatively slow growing, progressing over many years. Depending on your age, you may therefore never experience any serious symptoms as a result of your cancer. Treatment that is given before a cancer has spread is often effective, and your consultant should be able to give you some idea of the likely outcome in your case.

6. I have been diagnosed as having prostate cancer. Could my wife catch it by having sexual intercourse with me?

No - for two main reasons: women do not have prostate glands and cancer cannot be 'caught' from another person.

7. My father is due to have radiotherapy for prostate cancer. He has been told he will need treatment sessions every weekday for about 6 weeks. As it will be difficult for him to get to the hospital each day, is it possible for him to have one large dose of radiotherapy rather than several small ones?

Normal cells are able to repair themselves to some extent after smaller doses of radiation, whereas malignant cells are not and are gradually killed off. However, radiotherapy is rarely given in one large dose, as this would damage the normal tissue as well as the cancer cells.

Some hospitals and oncology centres have hostel wards where people who are in good health can stay each night during the week while they are undergoing treatment such as radiotherapy. People who stay in these hostels can come and go as they like, but are provided with meals and a bed at night. Your father could ask at his treatment centre if he can have a bed in a hostel ward so that he does not have to travel back and forth each day.

8. I have been told that after my prostate operation I will have to 'drink plenty' to help flush out my bladder. What sort of drinks should I have and how much is 'plenty'?

For the first couple of days after your operation you should try to drink up to 3 litres of clear fluid each day. Once the blood has cleared from your urine and you are able to urinate spontaneously again - which may take anything from 24 hours to several days - you can reduce your daily fluid intake to around 1.5 litres. Most types of drink are suitable, including water, tea, coffee, fruit juice and beer.

9. My father is waiting to have a radical prostatectomy. My mother is more or less dependent on his care, but will not agree to stay with me while he's in hospital, as I live too far away for her to be able to visit him. My parents are very independent, but I really don't think my mother will be able to manage alone. Is there anything I can do to make it possible for her to stay in her own home so she can visit my father in hospital every day?

You should be able to get help for your mother from your parents' local social services department. She will probably be entitled to 'meals on wheels' and a home help for as long as necessary - and your father too, once he's back at home after his operation. It is a good idea to work out exactly how much and what type of help your mother will need before you contact the social services, so that you can make sure that suitable arrangements are made for her.

10. I have recently started to have to get up three or four times a night to pass water. I also often need to urinate urgently during the day and sometimes can't stop urine leaking before I get to the toilet. Is it just my age (I am 58) and something I will have to put up with, or should I go to my doctor?

Your problems are likely to be associated with enlargement of your prostate gland, which *is* age related but not something you have to put up with. However, there could be other causes, including prostate cancer, and you should certainly see your doctor, who will probably refer you to a urology clinic for tests. The treatment you are given will depend on the diagnosis. If possible, make a note over the next few days of how often you urinate and any difficulties you have in passing urine and take it with you when you see your doctor.

11. Six weeks ago I had an operation to remove my prostate gland, but I still have almost the same problems as before -- needing to go to the toilet frequently both day and night and tending to leak urine before and after I urinate. Has the operation failed?

It can take several weeks or even months before the effects of prostate surgery become fully apparent, but your problems should gradually improve. Your bladder muscles have to regain their tone, and the operation itself can cause bruising and trauma to the urinary system. While you are waiting for your problems to resolve, it may be a good idea to buy some pads (from a pharmacy) to wear in your underpants to absorb any unavoidable urine leaks. A district nurse or a continence nurse at your hospital will be able to give you further advice.

The pelvic-floor exercises that you were probably told about while you were in hospital will also help you regain bladder control. However, incontinence after prostate surgery can occasionally be permanent and you should talk to your doctor if your problems persist, as investigations may need to be done to discover their cause.

12. I am waiting to have surgery for prostate cancer, but have recently begun to find passing urine painful and accompanied by a severe burning sensation in my penis. Should I go back to my doctor or just wait until I go into hospital - in about 5 weeks time?

It is important to tell your doctor about any change in your symptoms. You may have a urinary infection, which will need to be treated with antibiotics, or you may be starting to retain urine, in which case you may need to have a catheter inserted to drain your bladder.

13. I have been told I will probably have to stay in hospital for up to 7 days after my prostate operation, but I know someone who was discharged after only 3 days following prostate surgery. Why has such a long stay been anticipated for me?

Operations to reduce the size of the prostate gland, such as a transurethral resection, can be done through the urethra and therefore do not involve making an incision in the abdominal wall. Recovery from this type of surgery is usually relatively quick. Open and radical prostatectomies, on the other hand, involve making an incision in the abdomen, which will take time to heal. Also, these operations involve handling the bladder and bowel, which consequently take longer to return to normal function afterwards. It sounds as though your friend had a transurethral resection and that you require open surgery for prostate cancer. You should ask you doctor, consultant or a nurse specialist at the hospital to explain to you exactly what is going to happen during your operation.

14. I have prostate cancer for which I am receiving hormone therapy. However, I have heard that there is a new drug being tested that may be more effective than the drugs I am being given. I would like to take part in this drug trial. How do I go about it?

You can ask your doctor or consultant about the trial you mention and can certainly let them know that you would be interested in taking part. However, this particular trial may not include people in the area in which you live, or it may already have enough patients involved in it. You also have to bear in mind that some of the people involved in drug trials are given a placebo (which doesn't have any effect) or another drug that is being used as a comparison. So, even if you do take part in the trial, you cannot be sure that you will receive the drug you want.

15. I am due to have radiotherapy but would prefer to be given this treatment as brachytherapy, as I hear it may be more effective. Can I insist on having brachytherapy?

Brachytherapy is not widely available in the UK and therefore you probably won't be able to insist on having it. However, at present there is no evidence to suggest that it is *more* effective than external beam radiotherapy or radical surgery to remove the prostate gland, although it does have the advantage of avoiding the need to have to return regularly for treatment sessions.

16. I have advanced prostate cancer and am prepared to try any treatment that might cure it. I have heard that there's a new treatment called cryotherapy, but my doctor hasn't suggested I have this. Should I tell him I want it?

You should certainly talk to your doctor about all the treatment options, although, unfortunately, there is no treatment currently available that can cure advanced prostate cancer. Cryotherapy, for example, is only suitable for small cancers that have not extended beyond the capsule around the prostate gland. Any treatment you receive will be to deal with the symptoms you develop, rather than an attempt to cure your cancer. If you are still unsure about the various treatments available and their effects, it may be a good idea to ask to talk to a nurse specialist in more detail.

17. I've just been told that I have prostate cancer, but surely this can't be the case, as I had my prostate removed by transurethral resection some years ago?

Transurethral resection - and various similar operations - is done to remove *part* of an enlarged prostate gland that is causing urinary problems. The operation does not remove the entire prostate, and therefore the tissue that remains can still be affected by cancer. Many men have problems due to enlargement of their prostate glands as they get older, and their symptoms can be improved by surgery to reduce the size of the gland. Complete removal of the gland (prostatectomy) is only done if there is already cancer in it.

18. Is it true that eating a low-fat diet will cure my prostate cancer, which is at an early stage of development?

Although there is evidence to suggest (but not prove) that a diet high in animal fat increases the risk of developing prostate cancer, reducing the fat in your diet cannot cure it once it is already present. If you do need to have treatment, it will be in the form of radiotherapy, hormone therapy or surgery. However, eating a healthy, low-fat diet is always a good idea, and will certainly do no harm now.

19. Rather than have conventional treatment for my prostate cancer, I would like to explore alternative therapies. How effective are these?

Unfortunately, no alternative therapy has yet been proven to cure prostate cancer.

20. My father died from prostate cancer a few years ago, at the age of 65. What are my chances of developing it too and what can I do to reduce them?

There does seem to be a greater risk for men who have first-degree relatives with prostate cancer - perhaps up to three times greater than normal - although this depends on how many relatives are affected and the ages at which they developed the disease. However, there is no genetic test currently available that will tell you whether you have a gene that might make you more susceptible to prostate cancer. As the disease is fairly common in older men, your father may simply have been 'unlucky'.

However, you might be well-advised to have your prostate-specific antigen (PSA) level checked annually from the age of 45. A raised level at any time will alert your doctor to the need to do further tests to look for any signs of prostate cancer.

Otherwise, the advice for you is probably the same as that for any man: eat a healthy, low-fat diet and seek medical advice at the first sign of any urinary problems, as treatment at an early stage has more chance of being successful.

Appendix III

Medical terms

Adenocarcinoma A malignant tumour (cancer) of glandular epithelium. It is the most common type of prostate cancer.

Adjuvant therapy A treatment used in combination with another (primary) treatment to make it more effective.

Allergic reaction An abnormal reaction to a substance. An allergic reaction can be mild, causing an itchy rash, or severe, leading to fainting, vomiting, loss of consciousness or, rarely, death.

Anaesthesia The absence of sensation.

Anaesthetic A drug that causes loss of sensation in part or all of the body.

Anaesthetist A doctor trained in the administration of anaesthetics.

Analgesic A drug that blocks the sensation of pain; a painkiller.

Antibiotic A substance that kills bacteria or prevents them replicating.

Anticholinergic drug A drug that suppresses the action of acetylcholine, a chemical found in the tissues of the body that transmits nerve impulses at certain sites.

Anticoagulant A substance that prevents the blood from clotting.

Anti-embolism stockings Stockings that are sometimes worn during operations and post-operatively until the patient is able to move around again. They assist the circulation of blood in the legs and help to prevent blood clots forming. They are also sometimes called thrombo-embolic deterrent stockings, or TEDS.

Anti-emetic A drug that helps to reduce feelings of sickness.

Bacteraemia A condition caused by the presence of bacteria in the circulating blood.

Benign Non-malignant. A benign tumour will remain localized at its site of development and will have no harmful effect other than possibly to interfere with the function of nearby organs as it grows.

Benign prostatic hyperplasia The condition caused by enlargement of the prostate that occurs in men with age.

Biopsy The surgical removal of a piece of tissue from a living body for examination under a microscope to assist or confirm a diagnosis.

Bladder neck incision An operation that involves making a cut in the neck of the bladder or along the prostate gland to improve the symptoms of benign prostatic hyperplasia. It is sometimes the treatment of choice for a prostate gland that is not significantly enlarged.

Brachytherapy A new, and not yet widely available, treatment for delivering radioactivity to cancer cells in the prostate gland. It involves the insertion of either 'seeds'- **permanent seed brachytherapy** - or rods - **high-dose brachytherapy** - containing the radioactive material, which can destroy the cells of a cancer at an early stage of development.

Cancer A malignant growth resulting from the uncontrolled multiplication of cells that fail to die naturally. If left untreated, the cancer cells may invade nearby areas of the body and will eventually spread to distant sites.

Cannula A very fine tube or needle. Fluids can be introduced into or removed from the body through an intravenous cannula inserted into a vein, usually in the back of the hand. Anaesthetic drugs are administered through a cannula during an operation. Cannulae are usually made of plastic, but used to be metal or glass.

Carcinoma A cancer in epithelial tissue, such as that of the prostate gland or bladder. Carcinomas are always malignant, but their severity and tendency to spread can vary.

Catheter A thin tube used to withdraw fluid or introduce it into the body. Urinary catheters are usually inserted into the bladder via the urethra to drain the urine from it. Suprapubic catheters are inserted directly into the bladder through a small hole made in the lower abdominal wall.

Catheterization The insertion of a catheter.

Cauterize To burn a part with heat or some other agent. The severed ends of small blood vessels are sealed with the tip of an instrument heated by an electric current to stop them bleeding during surgery.

Chemotherapy Treatment with drugs.

Clinical nurse specialist A nurse with specialist knowledge who works closely with doctors and patients in a particular field of medicine and who is able to spend time talking to patients and answering their questions.

Complication A condition that occurs as the result of another disease or condition. It may also be an unwanted side effect of treatment.

Computerized tomography (CT) A scan that takes X-ray images through 'slices' of the body. The images are interpreted by a computer to build up a three-dimensional picture.

Connective tissue Fibrous tissue that connects and supports organs within the body.

Consent form A form that patients must sign before surgery to confirm that they understand what is involved in their operation and give their consent for it to take place. Signing the form also gives consent for the use of anaesthetic drugs and any other procedures that are felt to be necessary as surgery progresses.

Constipation Difficulty or infrequent opening of the bowels or retention of faeces. The condition can sometimes be relieved by a high-fibre diet or laxatives.

Consultant An experienced and fully trained doctor who specializes in a particular type of medicine.

Cryoprobe An instrument used in cryotherapy. It contains liquid nitrogen to freeze - and therefore kill - the cells of a prostate cancer. It is inserted through the rectum and guided into place using ultrasound scans.

Cryotherapy/Cryosurgery A treatment for prostate cancer that involves the use of liquid nitrogen to freeze the tissue of the tumour (at a temperature of -50°C or lower) and kill the cells. It is successful for small cancers that are still contained within the capsule surrounding the prostate gland. It is not yet widely available, nor is it known how effective it is in the long term.

Cyclo-oxygenase-2 (COX-2) inhibitors A new class of drugs that inhibit the activity of the enzyme cyclo-oxygenase-2, which is present in large amounts in cancer cells and which protects them from injury - including that caused by radiotherapy and chemotherapy.

Cystitis Inflammation of the bladder due to injury or infection.

Cystogram A series of X-rays taken after a dye has been inserted into the bladder. The X-rays are taken as the bladder empties and reveal any holes in the urethra through which urine is escaping.

Cystoscope A telescope-like surgical instrument with a light attached that can be inserted through the urethra to examine the bladder. Other instruments can be introduced through it as required.

Deep vein thrombosis (DVT) A blood clot in a deep vein, often in the lower leg or pelvis.

Defaecate To empty the bowels.

Detrusor decompensation Inability of the muscles of the bladder to contract properly, which causes the bladder to become floppy and unable to expel urine.

Detrusor instability Over-activity of the muscular layer of the bladder wall that causes the bladder to try to empty itself at inappropriate times. It can lead to symptoms such as frequency, urgency, nocturia and urge incontinence.

Diagnosis The identification of a disease based on its symptoms and signs.

Diarrhoea The frequent passage of unformed faeces.

Diathermy A method of generating heat by means of a high-frequency electric current. It is used in surgery to destroy diseased tissue or to stop bleeding from damaged blood vessels.

Discharge letter A letter that is given to patients leaving hospital (or sent directly from the hospital) to deliver to their family doctor giving details of the treatment they have had and of any necessary follow-up treatment they require.

Distant metastasis Spread of malignant cells via the blood or lymphatic vessels to sites that are distant from the primary cancer.

Diuretic A substance that increases the volume of urine produced.

Drain A tube, which may be attached to a bag or bottle, that is inserted near a wound to drain away excess blood and fluid.

Drip/Intravenous infusion A tube through which fluid is administered to replace that lost from the body after an operation or injury. One end is inserted into a vein in the arm and the other end is attached to a bottle or bag containing a specially balanced saline or sugar solution.

Efferent duct The duct that carries sperm from the seminiferous tubules in the testis to the epididymis.

Ejaculation The sudden ejection of semen from the penis following sexual arousal.

Ejaculatory duct The duct that carries semen from the seminal vesicle to the urethra in the penis.

Electrocardiogram (ECG) The activity of the heart recorded as a series of electrical wave patterns.

Electrocautery The application of the electrically heated tip of an instrument to the ends of blood vessels to stop them bleeding.

Embolus (plural: **emboli**) A piece of a blood clot (or air bubble) that has broken away and can pass through the blood vessels. If it lodges in a vital organ, such as the lung, it can have fatal consequences.

Epididymis A mass of tissue attached to the border of the testis that is made up of tightly coiled efferent ducts carrying sperm that have been produced in the testis.

Epidural anaesthetic An anaesthetic drug that is injected into the space around the nerves in the back. When used during an operation, it causes numbness in the legs and groin, which lasts for 3-5 hours. Epidurals can also be given continuously via a cannula to provide pain relief over several days.

Excision Removal by cutting.

Fertility In men, the capacity to induce conception; in women, the capacity to conceive and give birth. A man's fertility is dependent on the number and quality of his sperm and not on his ability to perform the sexual act.

Flow clinic A urology clinic at which various tests are done to investigate the cause of urinary symptoms.

Frequency (of micturition) The number of times the bladder needs to be emptied. Increased frequency can occur with various urinary and prostate conditions.

General anaesthetic A drug that induces loss of consciousness and abolishes the sensation of pain in all parts of the body.

Haematoma A blood-filled swelling. A haematoma can form after trauma or in a wound after an operation if blood continues to leak from a blood vessel. If the blood spreads in the tissues, it appears as a bruise.

Hemi-body radiotherapy Treatment to help relieve severe bone pain caused by the spread of advanced prostate cancer to the bones, which involves administering a single high dose of radiotherapy to half the body.

Heparin A substance that occurs naturally in the body and helps to prevent the blood clotting. It may be given in low doses by injection before and after surgery to people who are at particular risk of developing blood clots, for example during long periods of immobilization. Higher doses of heparin are given once a blood clot has formed to try to prevent it getting worse.

Hesitancy (of micturition) Difficulty in passing urine, which may result in a slow rate of flow.

Histological examination The examination under a microscope of a sample of tissue that has been taken from the body by biopsy.

Hormone therapy Treatment with drugs that affect the hormones which regulate the growth and function of organs. For example, drugs can be given to relieve the symptoms caused by a prostate cancer by suppressing the production of the hormone testosterone by the testes and thus slowing the rate of growth of the cancer.

Hospice A centre that provides medical care and various non-medical facilities for those with terminal illness and their families. Hospice staff help people to lead full and independent lives for as long as possible by giving them wide-ranging support, in some cases for many years.

Hostel ward A hospital ward set aside for people who do not need medical care but who are unable to go home immediately after an operation or between treatment sessions. Food and a bed are provided, but the ward does not have a full medical staff.

Hydronephrosis Dilatation of the drainage system of the kidneys that is caused by the accumulation of fluid and leads to enlargement of the kidneys themselves.

Hypertrophy Enlargement of an organ caused by an increase in the number and size of its cells.

Immunological treatment/Immunotherapy Treatment (usually involving the use of drugs) that activates the body's own immune mechanisms to fight disease.

Impotence The inability to get an erection. It is sometimes a side effect of prostate surgery.

Incision A cut or wound made by a sharp instrument, such as during an operation.

Incontinence The lack of voluntary control over the discharge of urine or faeces.

Induction agent A drug used in anaesthesia to induce loss of consciousness.

Inguinal canal A canal that runs from the abdomen, through the groin and into the scrotum and through which a testis descends in a male fetus before birth.

Inhalational anaesthetic An anaesthetic given as a mixture of gases that is inhaled, usually to maintain anaesthesia.

Intra-operative Occurring during an operation.

Intravenous anaesthetic A general anaesthetic drug that is injected into a vein via a cannula, usually in the back of the hand.

Intravenous pyelogram (IVP) An X-ray taken following the injection of a special dye into a vein in the arm. The dye enters the kidneys and is excreted via the ureters into the bladder.

Irritable bladder Over-activity of the muscles of the wall of the bladder, which causes it to try to empty at inappropriate times.

Keyhole surgery A colloquial name for laparoscopic surgery.

Laparoscopic surgery Surgery done with the aid of a telescope-like instrument called a laparoscope. The laparoscope has a light source and a camera attached to it and is introduced through a small hole in the body wall to enable the surgeon to examine the internal organs. Surgical instruments are inserted through similar small incisions. Because there is no large wound post-operatively, recovery time is reduced.

Laser treatment The destruction of tissue using lasers. The laser contains substances which, when stimulated by light energy, emit a beam of light of great intensity that can be directed precisely. Laser treatment can be used to destroy tissue from an enlarged prostate without causing bleeding.

Leakage of urine The dribbling of urine before or after urinating.

Lesion Any abnormality such as an injury, infection or tumour.

Libido Sexual desire.

Local anaesthetic An anaesthetic that numbs the area of the body around which it is injected.

Local injection An injection of a substance that remains confined to one area and is not distributed throughout the body.

Local metastasis Spread of malignant cells to the area immediately around the primary site of a cancer.

Lymph A pale-coloured fluid that flows within the lymphatic vessels of the body and is eventually returned to the blood. It contains disease-fighting cells, the lymphocytes.

Lymph node A gland through which lymph flows and is filtered and which acts as a store for the lymphocytes.

Lymphadenectomy Surgical removal of lymph nodes for examination when regional spread of cancer is suspected.

Lymphangiogram A test done to detect the spread of cancer to the lymph nodes. A special dye is injected into the lymphatic system, which highlights the lymph vessels and nodes on X-ray.

Lymphocyte A type of white blood cell involved in fighting disease in the body.

Magnetic resonance imaging (MRI) The use of a large magnet to produce a magnetic field in individual cells of the body. An energy field is applied that affects the alignment of atoms within the cells and causes them to emit a signal that is detected and interpreted as an image of the body.

Maintenance agent A drug used during an operation to maintain the state of general anaesthesia.

Malignant Used to describe a lesion that is likely to spread locally and to distant parts of the body - a cancer.

Metastasis (plural: **metastases**) A secondary cancer at a site distant from the original (primary) cancer.

Metastasis (verb: **metastasize**) The spread of cancerous cells through the blood or lymphatic vessels from the site of the original cancer.

Metastasize To spread to a distant part.

Metastatic disease Advanced cancer due to the spread of malignant cells from the primary tumour.

Microwave treatment The use of microwave radiation to destroy tissue selectively without causing bleeding. The treatment is sometimes used to remove tissue from an enlarged prostate gland, the instrument delivering the microwaves being inserted through the rectum or urethra.

Micturition The act of passing urine; urination.

Nasogastric tube A tube inserted via a nostril to drain the stomach and prevent vomiting. Nasogastric tubes are used after some types of operation or to feed patients who are unable to eat.

National Health Service (NHS) The system of medical care that was set up in Britain in 1948 to provide medical treatment that is mostly funded by taxation.

Nausea A feeling of sickness.

Neuroma A tumour of nerve cells and nerve fibres.

Nil by mouth A term used to mean that no food or drink should be swallowed in the hours before an operation.

Nocturia A condition that involves having to get up at night to pass urine (often small amounts) due to irritation of the bladder or a prostate problem.

Nocturnal polyuria The passage of large amounts of urine at night because the kidneys are producing more than they normally would.

Obesity An excessive amount of fat in the body. The term is non-specific and has now been replaced by a figure calculated from height and weight measurements, known as the **body mass index**.

Oncologist A physician specializing in the treatment of cancer.

Oncology The study and management of cancer.

Open prostatectomy Surgery to remove tissue from a very large prostate gland that is done through an incision made in the abdominal wall.

Orchidectomy Surgical removal of a testis. **Bilateral orchidectomy** (removal of both testes) is a type of hormone therapy that is sometimes undertaken to treat prostate cancer by reducing the level of testosterone on which the cancer depends.

Palliative therapy Treatment used to alleviate symptoms but which cannot cure the condition that is causing them.

Perineum The area of the body between the scrotum and anus.

Post-operative Following an operation.

Pre-medication ('pre-med.') A drug that is given before another drug, for example one given an hour or two before an operation to relax the patient before anaesthesia is started.

Pre-operative Before an operation.

Primary tumour The first (and sometimes only) or most important tumour to develop.

Prognosis An opinion about the probable course and final outcome of a disease that is made when all the known facts are considered.

Prophylaxis Preventative treatment.

Prostate gland The gland that surrounds the neck of the bladder and urethra in men and secretes a fluid that forms part of the semen. It often enlarges in elderly men, causing constriction of the urethra and thus urinary symptoms.

Prostate-specific antigen (PSA) A protein found in the blood of men, the level of which increases with various prostate diseases. It is significantly raised with prostate cancer.

Prostatectomy Surgical removal of part or all of the prostate gland.

Prostatism A syndrome caused by enlargement of the prostate gland that leads to urinary obstruction, and thus to retention of urine, hesitancy, urgency and nocturia.

Prostatitis Inflammation of the prostate gland that may or may not be due to bacterial infection but that can be treated with antibiotics. Its symptoms are similar to those of prostate enlargement.

Prostatotomy An operation done to relieve the symptoms caused by a slightly enlarged prostate. It involves making one or two cuts along the length of the prostate gland so that it falls away from the urethra, allowing urine to flow unobstructed.

Pulmonary embolism A blood clot or air bubble that blocks the blood vessels in the lung.

Pyrexia A fever.

Quality of life A person's general state of physical, functional, psychological and social well-being as compared to their own perceived normal state.

Radiation oncologist A radiotherapist.

Radical prostatectomy Surgical removal of the entire prostate gland, its capsule and the seminal vesicles. It involves making a long, vertical incision in the abdomen and is sometimes used to treat prostate cancer in its early stages of development.

Radical treatment Aggressive treatment aimed at curing a serious illness.

Radiographer A technician qualified in diagnostic imaging techniques.

Radiologist A doctor trained in diagnostic imaging.

Radiotherapist/Radiation oncologist A doctor specializing in the use of radiation as treatment, for example for cancer.

Radiotherapy Treatment with radiation.

Recovery room A ward near the operating theatre to which patients are taken after surgery so that they can be watched closely while they recover from a general anaesthetic.

Rectal examination The insertion of a finger through the rectum to feel the prostate gland.

Recurrence The reappearance of symptoms or signs of a disease after a period of apparent recovery.

Regional metastasis Spread of malignant cells to nearby sites, usually the nearest lymph nodes.

Regression The disappearance or reduction of the symptoms and signs of a disease.

Resectoscope A surgical instrument inserted through the urethra to cut away (resect) part of the prostate during transurethral resection.

Retention (of urine) The holding back of urine in the bladder due to obstruction or muscular weakness of the bladder wall. Acute retention can have serious consequences but can be relieved by the passage of a catheter, either through the urethra or suprapubically, to empty the bladder.

Retrograde ejaculation The passage of sperm back up the urethra into the bladder during ejaculation. It is a common side effect of prostate surgery and causes reduced fertility.

Scrotum A pouch of skin present in men that is divided into two by a septum, each half containing a testis, epididymis and the lower part of the spermatic cord.

Secondary tumour A tumour at a site distant from that of the original (primary) tumour; a metastasis.

Semen The fluid containing sperm and secretions from the prostate and seminal vesicles.

Seminal vesicle A coiled tube at the base of the bladder, adjacent to the prostate, which stores semen.

Seminiferous tubule A tube in the testis in which sperm are produced. Each testis contains one to three of these tightly coiled tubules.

Septicaemia Severe infection caused by large numbers of bacteria in the blood that multiply and spread.

Seroma A collection of clear fluid, such as lymph, which may develop following an operation. If persistent, the fluid can be drawn off with a needle.

Side effect An effect other than that desired, which results from the use of a drug or other form of treatment.

Sign Something a doctor looks for as an indication of disease, such as a lesion or swelling.

Sperm The mature male cell that contains male genetic material capable of developing into a new individual when united with a female egg. It consists of a small head region, a short middle piece, and a mobile tail that enables it to swim.

Spermatic cord The cord containing the nerves, blood and lymphatic vessels supplying the testis.

Spinal anaesthetic An anaesthetic that is injected between the vertebrae of the spine into the space around the nerves in the back. It causes numbness in the legs and groin, which lasts for 3-5 hours.

Staging Classification of the extent of a cancer, i.e. whether it is localized, has spread regionally or to distant sites in the body. The stage at which a cancer is first detected may have a bearing on the likely outcome of its treatment.

Stent A small coil or spiral that can be inserted into the top of the urethra to keep the sphincter into the bladder open and thus relieve obstruction. The use of stents is less effective than surgery and tends to be reserved for older men with urinary symptoms whose general health is poor.

Steroid One of a group of naturally occurring substances in the body that includes the sex hormones.

Strontium-89 A radioactive liquid that is sometimes used in the treatment of prostate cancer. It is injected into a vein, from where it is taken up by areas of bone affected by the spread of the disease. If the treatment is successful at relieving the bone pain, it can be repeated every 3-4 months. However, this type of treatment is not yet widely available.

Suture A surgical stitch or row of stitches.

Symptom Something experienced by a patient that indicates a disturbance of normal body function, for example pain or nausea.

Testis The male reproductive organ in which sperm develop; the testicle.

Testosterone The male sex hormone (a steroid) produced by the testes, which, amongst other things, plays a role in regulating the growth and function of the prostate.

Thrombo-embolic deterrent stockings (TEDS) *See* Anti-embolism stockings.

Thrombosis The coagulation of blood within a vein or artery that produces a blood clot.

Thrombus A blood clot that forms in, and remains in, a blood vessel or the heart.

Topical anaesthetic An anaesthetic that remains localized in the area in which it is applied.

Transrectal ultrasonography (TRUS) An ultrasound scan of the lower abdomen for which the scanning device is inserted into the rectum.

Transurethral resection of the prostate (TURP) The surgical removal of part of the prostate gland. The surgical instruments are introduced via the urethra and therefore the operation does not involve making an incision in the abdominal wall. The insertion of a small telescope allows the surgeon to view the organs and the operation as it progresses on a video or television monitor in the operating theatre.

Tumour A swelling; an abnormal growth of cells that can be benign or malignant. A **benign tumour** remains localized and does not spread to other parts of the body. It has no harmful effect, except possibly to compress adjacent organs as it enlarges. A **malignant tumour** (a cancer) will invade the surrounding tissues, interfering with their normal functioning. Cells from it may also spread to other parts of the body, giving rise to secondary tumours.

Ultrasonography *See* Ultrasound scan.

Ultrasound scan/Ultrasonography The passage of high-frequency sound waves through the body wall that are reflected back enabling an image of the internal organs to be built up by a computer.

Ureter The duct that transports urine from the kidney to the bladder.

Urethra The canal that carries urine from the bladder to the exterior. In men it also transports semen during ejaculation.

Urge incontinence The leakage of urine following a sudden need to urinate.

Urgency (of micturition) Difficulty controlling the sudden (and possibly frequent) need to pass urine.

Urinary incontinence Failure of the sphincter at the base of the bladder to close, leading to some degree of leakage of urine.

Urinary obstruction Obstruction of the bladder that prevents the free passage of urine through the urethra.

Urinary stasis The retention of a volume of urine in the bladder following urination.

Urine flow test Measurement of the volume and rate of flow of urine as it is passed into a funnel-shaped container attached to a meter.

Urodynamics Special tests to measure the pressures in the bladder and urethra to discover the cause of urinary symptoms. The tests are often done for people with incontinence and sometimes if obstruction by the prostate is suspected but not confirmed by other means. A tiny catheter is passed into the bladder, which is filled up. The pressures are measured while the bladder is filling and again when urine is passed. The tests may be combined with **video urodynamics**, which involves inserting a dye into the bladder and viewing it on a video screen as it empties.

Urologist A doctor with specific training in, and experience of, problems of the urinary system.

Vas deferens (plural: **vasa deferentia**) The tube that carries sperm from the testis to the penis.

Watchful waiting The regular monitoring of a condition that is causing mild to moderate symptoms. It may be appropriate for an older man with a small, slow-growing prostate cancer or for someone who is unfit for radical treatment.

X-ray A type of electromagnetic radiation of short wavelength that is able to pass through opaque bodies. It can be used in diagnosis, as it allows the internal structures and organs of the body to be seen. In higher doses it is used as therapy to destroy malignant cells.

Appendix IV

Useful addresses

There are organizations in every country that are able to provide information, practical advice and support to men with prostate cancer and to their families and friends. The alphabetical list below includes some in the UK and one or two national organizations for each of the other main English-speaking countries, all of which will make good starting points for anyone seeking further information and/or details of local support groups. Experienced cancer nurses are available to give confidential advice on most of the telephone helplines listed.

If you have access to the Internet, you will be able to find websites for other organizations around the world, for example by searching for 'prostate cancer' on one of the general information sites such as www.askjeeves.com or www.google.com.

CancerBACUP
3 Bath Place
Rivington Street
London EC2A 3JR
Telephone: 020 7739 2280
Helpline: 0808 800 1234 (weekdays 9 a.m.-7 p.m.)
Website: www.cancerbacup.org.uk

Cancer Care Society
11 The Cornmarket
Romsey
Hampshire SO51 8GB
Telephone: 01794 830 300
Website: details can be found on www.netdoctor.co.uk

Carers UK
20-25 Glasshouse Yard
Lower Crescent
London EC1A 4JT
Telephone: 020 7490 8818
Helpline: 0808 808 7777
Email: info@ukcarers.org
Website: www.carersonline.org.uk

CRUSE Bereavement Care
Cruse House
126 Sheen Road
Richmond
Surrey TW9 1UR
Telephone: 202 8939 9530
Helpline: 0870 167 1677
Email: info@crusebereavementcare.org.uk
Website: www.crusebereavementcare.org.uk

Institute for Complementary Medicine
PO Box 194
London SE16 7QZ
Telephone: 020 7237 5165
Email: icm@icmedicine.co.uk
Website: www.icmedicine.co.uk

Irish Cancer Society
5 Northumberland Road
Dublin 4
Ireland
Telephone: 01 2310 500
Helpline: 1 800 200 700 (weekdays 9.00 a.m.-4.30 p.m.)
Email: helpline@irishcancer.ie
Website: www.cancer.ie

Macmillan Cancer Relief
89 Albert Embankment
London SE1 7UQ
Telephone: 020 7840 7841
Helpline: 0808 808 2020 (weekdays 9 a.m.-6 p.m.)
Email: cancerline@macmillan.org.uk
Website: www.macmillan.org.uk

9 Castle Terrace
Edinburgh EH1 2DP
Telephone: 0131 229 3276

82 Eglantino Avonuo
Belfast BT9 6EU
Telephone: 02890 661166

Lloyds Bank Chambers
33 High Street, Cowbridge
South Glamorgan CF71 7AE
Telephone: 01446 775679

Marie Curie Cancer Care
89 Albcrt Embankment
London SE1 7TP
Telephone: 020 7599 7777
Email: info@mariecurie.org.uk
Website: www.mariecurie.org.uk

Prostate Cancer Charity
3 Angel Walk
Hammersmith
London W6 9HX
Telephone: 020 8222 7622
Helpline: 0845 300 8383 (weekdays 10 a.m.-4 p.m.)
Email: info@prostate-cancer.org.uk
Website: www.prostate-cancer.org.uk

Tak Tent Cancer Support Organisation (Scotland)
Flat 5
30 Shelley Court
Gartnavel Complex
Glasgow G12 0YN
Telephone: 0141 211 0122
Email: taktent@care4free.net
Website: www.taktent.org.uk

The Continence Foundation
307 Hatton Square
16 Baldwins Gardens
London EC1N 7RJ
Helpline: 0845 345 0165 (weekdays 9.30 a.m-12.30 p.m.)
Email: continence-help@dial.pipex.com
Website: www.continence-foundation.org.uk

The Ulster Cancer Foundation
40-42 Eglantine Avenue
Belfast BT9 6DX
Telephone: (028) 9066 3281
Helpline: 0800 783 33 39 (weekdays 9.00 a.m.-5.00 p.m.)
Email: info@ulstercancer.org
Website: www.ulstercancer.org

American Cancer Society
Telephone: 1-800-ACS-2345
Website: www.cancer.org

National Cancer Institute USA
NCI Public Inquiries Office
Sutie 3036A
6116 Executive Boulevard
MSC8322
Bethesda
MD 20892-8322
Helpline: 1-800-4-CANCER (1-800-422-6237)
Website: www.cancer.gov

National Prostate Cancer Coalition
1158 15th Street NW
Washington
DC 20005
Telephone: 202 463 9455
Toll-free: 888 245 9455
Email: info@pcacoalition.org
Website: www.pcacoalition.org

Australian Cancer Society/The Cancer Council Australia
GPO Box 4708
Sydney
NSW 2001
Telephone: 61 2 9380 9022
Cancer Information Service: 13 11 20
Email: info@cancer.org.au
Website: www.cancer.org.au

Canadian Cancer Society
National Office
Suite 200
10 Alcorn Avenue
Toronto
Ontario M4V 3BI
Telephone: 416 961 7223
Email: info@cis.cancer.ca
Website: www.cancer.ca

Cancer Society of New Zealand
PO Box 10847
Wellington
Telephone: 64 4 494 7270
Email: admin@cancernz.org.nz
Website: www.cancernz.org.nz

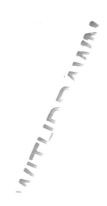